INTERVENTIONAL CARDIOLOGY CLINICS

www.interventional.theclinics.com

Editor-in-Chief

MATTHEW J. PRICE

Left Atrial Appendage Closure

April 2018 • Volume 7 • Number 2

Editor

APOSTOLOS TZIKAS

ELSEVIER

1600 John F. Kennedy Boulevard • Suite 1800 • Philadelphia, Pennsylvania, 19103-2899

http://www.theclinics.com

INTERVENTIONAL CARDIOLOGY CLINICS Volume 7, Number 2
April 2018 ISSN 2211-7458, ISBN-13: 978-0-323-58310-7

Editor: Lauren Boyle
Developmental Editor: Donald Mumford

Interventional Cardiology Clinics (ISSN 2211-7458) is published quarterly by Elsevier Inc., 360 Park Avenue South, New York, NY 10010-1710. Months of issue are January, April, July, and October. Subscription prices are USD 195 per year for US individuals, USD 449 for US institutions, USD 100 per year for US students, USD 195 per year for Canadian individuals, USD 536 for Canadian institutions, USD 150 per year for Canadian students, USD 295 per year for international individuals, USD 536 for international institutions, and USD 150 per year for international students. To receive student/resident rate, orders must be accompanied by name of affiliated institution, date of term, and the *signature* of program/residency coordinator on institution letterhead. Orders will be billed at individual rate until proof of status is received. Foreign air speed delivery is included in all *Clinics* subscription prices. All prices are subject to change without notice. **POSTMASTER:** Send address changes to *Interventional Cardiology Clinics*, Elsevier Health Sciences Division, Subscription Customer Service, 3251 Riverport Lane, Maryland Heights, MO 63043. **Customer Service: Telephone: 1-800-654-2452** (U.S. and Canada); **1-314-447-8871** (outside U.S. and Canada). **Fax: 1-314-447-8029. E-mail: journalscustomerservice-usa@elsevier.com (for print support); journalsonlinesupport-usa@elsevier.com (for online support).**

Reprints. For copies of 100 or more of articles in this publication, please contact the Commercial Reprints Department, Elsevier Inc., 360 Park Avenue South, New York, NY 10010-1710. Tel.: 212-633-3874; Fax: 212-633-3820; E-mail: reprints@elsevier.com.

CONTRIBUTORS

EDITOR-IN-CHIEF

MATTHEW J. PRICE, MD
Director, Cardiac Catheterization Laboratory, Division of Cardiovascular Diseases, Scripps Clinic, Assistant Professor, Scripps Translational Science Institute, La Jolla, California, USA

EDITOR

APOSTOLOS TZIKAS, MD, PhD
Department of Cardiology, AHEPA University Hospital of Thessaloniki, Interbalkan European Medical Centre, Thessaloniki, Greece

AUTHORS

SAMUEL J. ASIRVATHAM, MD
Professor, Medicine and Pediatrics, Departments of Pediatric Cardiology and Cardiovascular Diseases, Mayo Clinic Rochester, Rochester, Minnesota, USA

IGNACIO CRUZ-GONZALEZ, MD, PhD
Professor, Cardiology Department, University Hospital of Salamanca, Biomedical Research Institute of Salamanca (IBSAL), CIBER-CV, Salamanca, Spain

TAWSEEF DAR, MD
Cardiac Arrhythmia Fellow, Division of Cardiovascular Diseases, Cardiovascular Research Institute, University of Kansas Hospital and Medical Center, Kansas City, Kansas, USA

DAVID B. DELURGIO, MD, FACC, FHRS
Professor, Medicine, Emory University School of Medicine, Director, Electrophysiology, Emory St Joseph's Hospital, Atlanta, Georgia, USA

ABDALLAH EL SABBAGH, MD
Department of Cardiovascular Diseases, Mayo Clinic Rochester, Rochester, Minnesota, USA

MARVIN H. ENG, MD
Structural Heart Disease Fellowship Program Director, Center for Structural Heart Disease, Henry Ford Hospital, Detroit, Michigan, USA

THOMAS A. FOLEY, MD
Assistant Professor, Radiology, Departments of Diagnostic Radiology and Cardiovascular Diseases, Mayo Clinic Rochester, Rochester, Minnesota, USA

THOMAS J. FORBES, MD
Director, Cardiac Catheterization Laboratory, Assistant Professor, Pediatrics, Carmen and Ann Adams Department of Pediatrics, Children's Hospital of Michigan, Pediatric Cardiology, Wayne State University School of Medicine, Detroit, Michigan, USA

MONICA FUERTES-BARAHONA, MD
Cardiology Department, University Hospital of Salamanca, Biomedical Research Institute of Salamanca (IBSAL), CIBER-CV, Salamanca, Spain

ROCIO GONZALEZ-FERREIRO, MD
Cardiology Department, University Hospital of Salamanca, Biomedical Research Institute of Salamanca (IBSAL), CIBER-CV, Salamanca, Spain

DAVID R. HOLMES Jr, MD
Department of Cardiovascular Diseases, Mayo Clinic College of Medicine, Mayo Clinic, Rochester, Minnesota, USA

MICHAEL H. HOSKINS, MD
Associate Professor, Medicine, Emory University School of Medicine, Emory University Hospital, Atlanta, Georgia, USA

REDA IBRAHIM, MD
Department of Medicine, Montreal Heart Institute, Université de Montréal, Montreal, Québec, Canada

JESPER MØLLER JENSEN, MD, PhD
Department of Cardiology, Aarhus University Hospital, Aarhus N, Denmark

KASPER KORSHOLM, MD
Department of Cardiology, Aarhus University Hospital, Aarhus N, Denmark

DHANUNJAYA LAKKIREDDY, MD, FACC, FHRS
Professor, Medicine, Division of Cardiovascular Diseases, Cardiovascular Research Institute, University of Kansas Hospital and Medical Center, Kansas City, Kansas, USA

YAN YIN LAM, MD
Cardiology Department, Centre Medical, Hong Kong, China

GEORGE G. LATUS, BSBME
Boston Scientific, St Paul, Minnesota, USA

JAMES C. LEE, MD
Center for Structural Heart Disease, Henry Ford Hospital, Detroit, Michigan, USA

BERNHARD MEIER, MD
Professor, Department of Cardiology, University Hospital of Bern, Bern, Switzerland

NATHAN MESSAS, MD
Department of Medicine, Montreal Heart Institute, Université de Montréal, Montreal, Québec, Canada; Department of Cardiology, University Hospital of Strasbourg, Strasbourg, France

JOSE C. MORENO-SAMOS, MD
Cardiology Department, University Hospital of Salamanca, Biomedical Research Institute of Salamanca (IBSAL), CIBER-CV, Salamanca, Spain

JENS ERIK NIELSEN-KUDSK, MD, DMSc
Professor, Department of Cardiology, Aarhus University Hospital, Aarhus N, Denmark

HEYDER OMRAN, MD
Professor, Department of Cardiology, GFO Kliniken Bonn, Bonn, Germany

ANSHUL M. PATEL, MD, FACC, FHRS
Assistant Professor, Medicine, Emory University School of Medicine, Director, Arrhythmia Center, Emory St Joseph's Hospital, Atlanta, Georgia, USA

MATTHEW J. PRICE, MD
Director, Cardiac Catheterization Laboratory, Division of Cardiovascular Diseases, Scripps Clinic, Assistant Professor, Scripps Translational Science Institute, La Jolla, California, USA

PEDRO L. SANCHEZ, MD, PhD
Professor, Cardiology Department, University Hospital of Salamanca, Biomedical Research Institute of Salamanca (IBSAL), CIBER-CV, Salamanca, Spain

JACQUELINE SAW, MD
Clinical Professor, Interventional Cardiology, Program Director, Interventional Cardiology Fellowship Training Program, Vancouver General Hospital, University of British Columbia, Vancouver, British Columbia, Canada

ROBERT S. SCHWARTZ, MD
Director, Advanced Imaging Research, Minneapolis Heart Institute, Minneapolis, Minnesota, USA

SETH H. SHELDON, MD, FACC
Clinical Assistant Professor, Medicine, Division of Cardiovascular Diseases, Cardiovascular Research Institute, University of Kansas Hospital and Medical Center, Kansas City, Kansas, USA

HORST SIEVERT, MD
Professor, Cardiovascular Center Frankfurt CVC, Frankfurt, Germany

WIM STEGINK, MBA
Abbott, Coordination Center, Corporate Village, Zaventem, Belgium

FREDERIKE STOCK
Department of Cardiology, GFO Kliniken Bonn, Bonn, Germany

ALAN SUGRUE, MB, BCh, BAO
Department of Cardiovascular Diseases, Mayo
Clinic Rochester, Rochester, Minnesota, USA

NICHOLAS Y. TAN, MD, MS
Department of Internal Medicine, Mayo Clinic
Rochester, Rochester, Minnesota, USA

MOHMAD TANTARY, MD
Hospitalist, Department of Internal Medicine,
Clinch Valley Medical Center, Richlands,
Virginia, USA

JAY THAKKAR, MBBS, MD
Vancouver General Hospital, University of
British Columbia, Vancouver, British
Columbia, Canada; The George Institute for
Global Health, Camperdown, New South
Wales, Australia; The University of Sydney,
Broadway, New South Wales, Australia

MOHIT K. TURAGAM, MD
Cardiac Electrophysiology Fellow, Division of
Cardiology, Helmsey Center for
Electrophysiology, Icahn School of Medicine
at Mount Sinai, New York, New York, USA

APOSTOLOS TZIKAS, MD, PhD
Department of Cardiology, AHEPA University
Hospital, Interbalkan European Medical
Centre, Thessaloniki, Greece

ROBERT A. VAN TASSEL, MD
Minneapolis Heart Institute Foundation,
Minneapolis, Minnesota, USA

DIMITRA VASDEKI, MD
AHEPA University Hospital, Thessaloniki,
Greece

DEE DEE WANG, MD, FACC, FASE,
FSCCT
Director, Structural Heart Imaging, Medical
Director, 3D Printing, Henry Ford
Innovations Institute, Clinical Assistant
Professor, Wayne State University School of
Medicine, Center for Structural Heart
Disease, Henry Ford Hospital, Detroit,
Michigan, USA

BHARATH YARLAGADDA, MD
Cardiac Arrhythmia Fellow, Division of
Cardiovascular Diseases, Cardiovascular
Research Institute, University of Kansas
Hospital and Medical Center, Kansas City,
Kansas, USA

OMAR Z. YASIN, MD, MS
Department of Internal Medicine, Mayo
Clinic Rochester, Rochester, Minnesota,
USA

CONTENTS

Percutaneous left atrial appendage occlusion was introduced as an alternative method for prevention of thromboembolism in patients with nonvalvular atrial fibrillation after extensive animal work in 2001. The first device was named Percutaneous Left Atrial Appendage Transcatheter Occlusion (PLAATO) and patented by the company Appriva. The device was invented by Michael Lesh, MD.

A new era in antiembolic therapy has been initiated by the growing numbers of device-based therapies. Early concerns surrounding eliminating this enigmatic structure have not proven true. Other benefits are being further evaluated. Many other questions remain, such as whether there is a device-specific outcome effect or whether it is a class effect. Other questions include other devices, what head-to-head studies will show, and the impact of residual leak. Left atrial appendage using the Watchman ablation strategy can reduce cardioembolic stroke, with comparable or fewer adverse effects by device technology than obtained by long-term anticoagulation with its attendant bleeding risks.

AMPLATZER devices preceded WATCHMAN occluder in 2002 for catheter-based left atrial appendage occlusion. The AMPLATZER technique facilitates simultaneous closure of atrial shunts using 2 devices through 1 gear. Randomized WATCHMAN follow-up data showed a mortality benefit over warfarin. AMPLATZER data make this likely valid for the strategy. Particularly young people with atrial fibrillation should be offered left atrial appendage occlusion because the risk is confined to the intervention and early postintervention period. Guidelines should be adapted to make this progress in prevention of stroke and bleeding in patients with atrial fibrillation accessible for all, in the sense of a mechanical vaccination.

Resection of the left atrial appendage (LAA) to prevent recurrent arterial emboli in patients with atrial fibrillation was first suggested more than 60 years ago. Longer-term follow-up from randomized studies of the safety and efficacy of transcatheter LAA occlusion has recently been completed; data from large, observational cohorts are being reported. These recent data provide further insights into procedural safety with current techniques and the ability of LAA closure to reduce thromboembolic stroke compared with warfarin anticoagulation. This article summarizes the latest data regarding transcatheter LAA occlusion, focusing on larger prospective studies and further analyses of seminal clinical trials.

Left atrial appendage closure (LAAC) has emerged as a viable option for stroke prevention, especially in those intolerant of or not suitable for long-term oral anticoagulation therapy. This article describes the clinical characteristics, indications, and a proposed referral system for potential LAAC patients. Patient selection remains a challenge because of the paradox between the available randomized data on this intervention and the actual patient population that may gain maximum benefit. Further investigations comparing different LAAC devices with each other and with novel oral anticoagulants are needed. Also, the optimal antithrombotic regimen post-procedure has yet to be determined.

The left atrial appendage has been implicated as a major nidus for thrombus formation, particularly in atrial fibrillation. This discovery has prompted substantial interest in the development of left atrial appendage exclusion devices aimed at decreasing systemic thromboembolism risk. Its deceptively simple appearance belies the remarkable complexity that characterizes its anatomy and physiology. We highlight the key anatomic features and variations of the left atrial appendage as well as its relationships with surrounding structures. We also summarize crucial anatomic factors that should be taken into account by the interventional cardiologist when planning for or performing left atrial appendage exclusion procedures.

Randomized clinical trials have demonstrated that left atrial appendage (LAA) closure with the WATCHMAN device provides stroke prevention in nonvalvular atrial fibrillation while significantly reducing morality and major bleeding. Technical and procedural considerations are paramount for the therapeutic success. Maximizing procedural safety is critical. Optimal LAA sealing is required. Improvements in procedural technique and operator training have resulted in a marked reduction in adverse procedural events, which should increase the absolute long-term clinical benefit. This article outlines the key aspects of patient workup and procedural technique for the best possible outcome.

Percutaneous left atrial appendage occlusion (LAAO) for stroke prevention in patients with atrial fibrillation has significantly advanced in the past 2 decades. LAAO has emerged as a feasible and safe alternative to oral anticoagulants in patients who are deemed high risk for bleeding or are ineligible to receive anticoagulation. Herein, the authors review the main design features of the AMPLATZER Amulet device and describe step-by-step technical considerations for implantation of this LAAO device.

Left atrial appendage occlusion (LAAO) is a rapidly evolving technology. Multi-modality imaging and understanding of left atrial appendage anatomy are sure to advance. Two-dimensional and 3-dimensional transesophageal echocardiography with fluoroscopy are the mainstay for LAAO image-guided therapy. Key to successful LAAO is an understanding of the transseptal puncture, LAAO size selection for the device-specific landing zone, and postdeployment evaluation for leak and complications. With advancements in computed tomography, there may be a greater role for intracardiac echocardiographic imaging in specific types of LAAO anatomy and devices.

 Video content accompanies this article at http://www.interventional.theclinics.com.

Transcatheter left atrial appendage occlusion is increasingly used for stroke prevention in atrial fibrillation. The technique has proven effective and safe in randomized trials and multiple observational studies. The procedure is challenging due to the complex anatomy of the left atrial appendage; accurate cardiac imaging is essential for procedural guidance. Transesophageal echocardiography is the gold standard, but cardiac computed tomography (CT) has gained increasing interest in recent years. Cardiac CT offers high-resolution imaging allowing for preprocedural anatomic evaluation and device sizing, but also may be useful for exclusion of left atrial appendage thrombus, and follow-up assessment of residual peri-device leaks.

Major procedural complications related to left atrial appendage occlusion (LAAO) are relatively infrequent but may be associated with major morbidity and mortality. LAAO operators should be knowledgeable about these potential complications. Prompt recognition and treatment are necessary to avoid rapid deterioration and dire consequences. With stringent guidelines on operator training, competency requirements, and procedural-technical refinements, LAAO can be performed safely with low complication rates. This article focuses on commonly used devices, as well as prevention, treatment, and management of complications of LAAO.

Since the first percutaneous left atrial appendage occlusion (LAAO), many studies have shown the safety and efficacy of this technique to prevent embolic strokes in nonvalvular atrial fibrillation. The design, characteristics, and clinical data of the most frequently used devices for LAAO are reviewed, including the Amplatzer cardiac plug and Amulet (Abbott Vascular), the Watchman (Boston Scientific), and the LARIAT device (SentreHEART). Similarly, newer closer devices, such as Ultraseal (Cardia), LAmbre (Lifetech), and Coherex WaveCrest (Johnson & Johnson), also are discussed. Finally, new technologies still in the stage of preclinical study or in the initial clinical experience also are reviewed.

The epidemic of atrial fibrillation (AF) requires a comprehensive management strategy that uses the full force of available data and technology, including anti-coagulation, ablative therapy, and left atrial appendage occlusion. Patient-centered care with an emphasis on shared decision-making is particularly relevant to the authors' understanding of the complexity of AF and has helped them tailor therapy in this ever-growing patient population.

LEFT ATRIAL APPENDAGE CLOSURE

THE CLINICS ARE NOW AVAILABLE ONLINE!

Access your subscription at:
www.theclinics.com

PREFACE

Left Atrial Appendage Occlusion for Stroke Prevention in Patients with Atrial Fibrillation

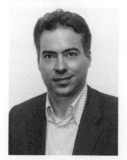

Apostolos Tzikas, MD, PhD
Editor

Percutaneous left atrial appendage (LAA) occlusion aims to address an important clinical need for patients with atrial fibrillation (AF): effective protection against thromboembolism without bleeding events. Finding the fine balance between *unnecessary* thrombus formation that may embolize and cause cerebral or other organ ischemia and *necessary* thrombus formation that protects against bleeding has been a challenge for all systemic medical therapies. Hence, human coagulation physiology is not yet modifiable and thrombosis is not always such a bad thing to happen; occasionally it is lifesaving. Therefore, the time may have come to consider "local therapy" against AF-related thromboembolism, with device closure of the LAA and less or no use of antithrombotic drugs. In this special issue of *Interventional Cardiology Clinics*, we present a series of articles written by world experts in the field, who cover the most relevant topics related to this intervention.

Starting with the history of percutaneous LAA occlusion, we asked some of the pioneers in the field, like Horst Sievert, David Holmes, Bernhard Meier, and Heyder Omran, to describe their part of the story. In the first three articles of this issue, the rationale, initial manufacturing steps, and a few personal details about PLATOO, WATCHMAN, and AMPLATZER devices are shared, many of which for the first time in the literature. Next, Dr Matthew Price summarizes the most important available clinical data in the field, and Tawseef Dar and colleagues discuss the indications and referral pathways for the quite heterogeneous patient population that could benefit from LAA closure. Nicholas Tan and colleagues wrote a comprehensive review on the anatomic and physiologic roles of the LAA, focusing on endocardial and epicardial device closure. Technical considerations and a stepwise procedural approach for the most widely used LAA occluders, the WATCHMAN, and the AMPLATZER AMULET device, are presented by Dr Matthew Price and Dr Messas and colleague, respectively. Cardiac imaging is fundamental for LAA closure therapy, mainly due to the high anatomical variability of the appendage. The use of echocardiography, with practical tips and tricks, is explained by Dr Wang and colleagues, and Dr Korsholm and colleagues provides a comprehensive review of the use of cardiac CT for LAA closure. In another article that provides practical insights,

Intervent Cardiol Clin 7 (2018) xiii–xiv
https://doi.org/10.1016/j.iccl.2018.01.002
2211-7458/18/© 2018 Published by Elsevier Inc.

Dr Thakkar and colleagues review the incidence, prevention, and management of the most common complications of LAA occlusion. The current landscape of LAA occluders that are in different phases of development together with a glimpse into the future of LAA closure technology is discussed by Dr Cruz-Gonzalez and colleagues. Last but not least, Dr Hoskins and colleagues wrote a very interesting article about the shared decision making and comprehensive management of patients with AF.

I would like to thank all the authors for their valuable contribution to this special issue.

Apostolos Tzikas, MD, PhD
AHEPA University Hospital of Thessaloniki &
Interbalkan European Medical Centre
Kiriakidi 1
Thessaloniki 54637, Greece

E-mail address:
aptzikas@yahoo.com

A History of Percutaneous Left Atrial Appendage Occlusion with the PLAATO Device

Heyder Omran, MD[a],*, Apostolos Tzikas, MD, PhD[b],
Horst Sievert, MD[c], Frederike Stock[a]

KEYWORDS

- Left atrial appendage • PLAATO • Atrial fibrillation • Left atrial appendage occlusion

KEY POINTS

- Percutaneous left atrial appendage occlusion was introduced as an alternative method for prevention of thromboembolism in patients with nonvalvular atrial fibrillation after extensive animal work in 2001.
- The first device was named Percutaneous Left Atrial Appendage Transcatheter Occlusion (PLAATO) and was invented by Michael Lesh, MD.

INTRODUCTION

Atrial fibrillation is the most common arrhythmia in adults and is associated with an increased mortality.[1] Thromboembolism is the most feared complication in patients with permanent atrial fibrillation.[2] The risk of embolism may vary from less than 1% to 20% depending on the underlying disease of the patient.[3] Patients with previous strokes have the highest risk of embolism. Transesophageal echocardiographic studies show that most thrombi are located in the left atrial appendage (LAA) and only few thrombi originate in the left atrium itself.[4,5] Although prospective and randomized studies show that oral anticoagulation (OAC) reduces the risk of thromboembolism significantly,[6] patients often may not receive OAC due to bleeding complications, increased bleeding risk, allergies to oral anticoagulants, or fear of complications.[7]

In 2001, an alternative procedure was introduced for patients with contraindications for OAC, that is, the interventional occlusion of the LAA.[8] This article provides information on the development, application, and results of this new technique.

IMAGING OF THE LEFT ATRIAL APPENDAGE

A prerequisite for the understanding of the mechanism of thromboembolism in patients with atrial fibrillation was adequate imaging of cardiac structures, in particular of the left atrium. In 1986, Aschenberg and colleagues[9] reported the detection of LAA thrombus by the use of transesophageal echocardiography. Further development of transesophageal echocardiographic imaging technology with higher-resolution and multiplane imaging allowed even better imaging of the LAA and understanding of its morphology and function.[10] In 1993, Flachskampf and colleagues[11] reported the initial experiences with a multiplanar transesophageal echoscope and outlined the usefulness for evaluating the LAA. The authors and other

[a] Department of Cardiology, GFO Kliniken Bonn, Robert-Koch-Str. 1, Bonn 53115, Germany; [b] Department of Cardiology, AHEPA University Hospital, Kiriakidi 1 Street, Thessaloniki 54637, Greece; [c] Cardiovascular Center Frankfurt CVC, Seckbacher Landstraße 65, Frankfurt 60389, Germany
* Corresponding author.
E-mail address: heyder.omran@marien-hospital-bonn.de

Intervent Cardiol Clin 7 (2018) 137–142
https://doi.org/10.1016/j.iccl.2017.12.009
2211-7458/18/© 2017 Elsevier Inc. All rights reserved.

investigators used imaging technology to assess the significance of LAA morphology and function in atrial fibrillation prior to cardioversion.[12]

In 1996, Dr Omran met Michael Lesh, the inventor of PLAATO in Königswinter, Germany, in Bonn, Germany, on a symposium arranged by Bernd Lüderitz, the head of the Department of Cardiology, University of Bonn. Michael Lesh presented the development of an interventional technology for percutaneous ablation of atrial fibrillation. Michael Lesh knew of the importance of the LAA for thromboembolism and thought of occluding the LAA using a percutaneous interventional approach.

PATENT OF A LEFT ATRIAL OCCLUSION DEVICE

In 1998, a patent on a device for LAA occlusion was issued by the company Appriva Medical (Sunnyvale, CA), founded by Michael Lesh (patent number US 6152144) (Please note, Appriva Medical Inc, is no longer operational and the original device is no longer being sold or produced).[13] The patent describes a "device and method for obliterating or occluding a body cavity or passageway, in particular, the LAA of a patient's heart. The procedure can be carried out intraoperatively, but is preferably carried out percutaneously by use of a delivery catheter to position an occluding device adjacent a patient's LAA. The occluding device may prevent the passage of embolic or other material to or from the LAA by volumetrically filling the appendage, closing the opening of the appendage with an occluding member, or pulling the tissue around the opening of the appendage together and fixing it in a closed state."

DEVICE DESCRIPTION

The device was called Percutaneous Left Atrial Appendage Transcatheter Occlusion (PLAATO). It consisted of a self-expanding balloon-shaped nitinol cage with multiple struts that produce an outward force. The diameter ranged from 15 mm to 32 mm. The frame itself was produced by laser-cutting a single tube of nitinol. Thereafter it was formed and heat-set to a self-expanding cage. The cage was partly covered with an occlusive expanded polytetrafluoroethylene (ePTFE) membrane (Fig. 1). The membrane covered the atrial surface of the device, whereas the opposite surface was not covered, allowing secondary thrombosis of the lumen by the device. Three rows of small anchors penetrated the membrane and were used to stabilize

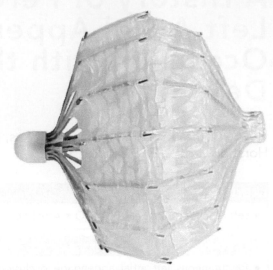

Fig. 1. An example of the first LAA occlusion device. It consists of a self-expanding balloon-shaped nitinol cage with an expanded ePTFE membrane with 3 rows of anchors.

the device in the appendage. A specifically designed 12F delivery catheter allowed for percutaneous implantation of the device itself and to inject contrast dye both distal and proximal to the device. The device could be collapsed and retrieved within the delivery catheter and repositioned in the LAA. Furthermore, the occlusion system enabled complete removal and replacement of the device. The device itself was locked with a string. After removal of the string, the device was unlocked and could be permanently implanted (Figs. 2–4).

ANIMAL STUDIES

Apart from intensive bench work, systematic animal studies were performed. In 2002, Nakai and colleagues[14] published the results of their animal work in *Circulation*. The investigators

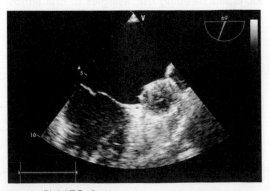

Fig. 2. PLAATO device.

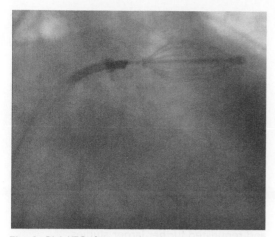

Fig. 3. PLAATO device within the LAA unexpanded.

successfully implanted the PLAATO device in a total of 25 dogs. The procedure times ranged from 45 minutes to 125 minutes and averaged 73 minutes ± 19 minutes. The device size was based on oversizing the diameter of the LAA by 20% to 40%. The final implanted device diameter ranged from 17 mm to 29 mm, which was 22% to 54% larger than the measured LAA diameters. The mean residual compression, hence, was 14%. They observed no major complications, apart from 1 small pericardial effusion. Device migration or dislodgment was not observed by intracardiac echocardiography or contrast fluoroscopy. Mitral valve function and pulmonary

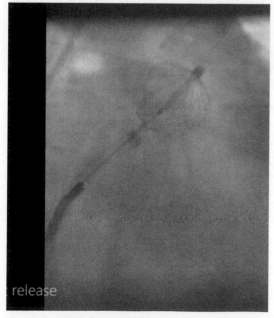

release

Fig. 4. PLAATO device about to be released.

vein inflow were not impaired and no thrombus was detected on the device during the procedure.

A total of 6 dogs were followed for 6 month to 1 year. Dislodgment was not observed and imaging confirmed occlusion of the devices.

Gross examination and histologic assessment showed that the devices were stable in the LAA in all cases. Macroscopic evidence of tissue attachment around the edges of the implant were already seen after 1 month. Complete healing over the membrane surface by an organized neointima and incorporation of the device in the attached walls was observed after 3 months.

Thrombus formation was not found, even with scanning electron microscopy in 5 animals.

FIRST IN HUMANS

In 2000, Michael Lesh asked a group of investigators to evaluate the feasibility and safety of the PLAATO device in humans with a contraindication for permanent OAC. In August 2001, Horst Sievert performed the first successful implantation of the PLAATO device in Frankfurt, Germany. One month later, the authors' study group implanted the second PLAATO device successfully in the first female patient at the University of Bonn.[15]

The results on the first 15 patients were reported in 2002 in *Circulation*.[8] LAA occlusion with the PLAATO device was successful in all patients. The first patient had hemopericardium during the first attempt, however, and the procedure had to be repeated after 30 days, highlighting the most feared complication of LAA occlusion. All procedures were guided by transesophageal echocardiography. After transseptal access, angiography was performed and according to instructions the size of the LAA determined. In concordance with previous animal work, a device was chosen that had a diameter at least greater than 20% larger than the diameter of the LAA landing zone. All patients were heparinized, aiming at an activated clotting time (ACT) greater than 250 seconds. The delivery catheter was used to approach the LAA. Thereafter, the device was realized and positioned in the neck of the LAA to completely occlude the os. Radiocontrast was injected distally and proximally to the device to control for location and adherence to adjacent tissue and assess sealing of the LAA. If no leaks were found and the location was appropriate, stability of the device was tested by gently pulling on the device. If all criteria were met, the device was released. Otherwise the device was collapsed, repositioned, and re-expanded. If the size of the device was inadequate, the device itself was recaptured and replaced by a new device. All patients received acetylic acid, 300 mg per day, indefinitely. In addition, patients received clopidogrel, 75 mg per day, for 6 months.

The median size of the final implanted device was 26 mm, ranging from 18 mm to 32 mm. The mean procedure time was 93 minutes. In 4 of 15 patients the device had to be replaced. During the follow-up of 1 month there were no late complications, embolic events, or migration of the devices. In addition, transesophageal echocardiography showed smooth healing of the surface of the device without thrombus formation.

INTERNATIONAL MULTICENTER STUDIES

After initial successful implantation of the PLAATO device, 2 concurrent prospective feasibility studies were conducted, 1 in Europe and 2 in North America.[16] The purpose of these studies, which had been published together, was to evaluate the feasibility and the safety of the device in a larger cohort of patients with nonrheumatic atrial fibrillation who were either on very high risk for ischemic stroke or were contraindicated to long-term OAC. Enrollment started in 2001 and finished in November 2003. Major adverse events (ie, stroke, myocardial infarction, and cardiac or neurologic death) and requirement for cardiovascular surgery related to the PLAATO procedure were the primary endpoints of the studies. Secondary endpoints were the ability of the PLAATO device to occlude the LAA and to avoid major adverse events during the initial hospitalization period. Device performance was also assessed as implantation success and treatment success. Patients with thrombus formation in the left atrial cavity, including the appendage; mitral or aortic stenosis or regurgitation; a left atrial diameter greater than 65 mm; and recent stroke were excluded from the study. Antiplatelet therapy consisted of acetylic acid and clopidogrel.

PLAATO was successful in 108 of 111 attempted patients. The average procedure time was 68 minutes. Clinical follow-up after 6 months was 90% and 69% after 1 year. One of 111 patients had 2 major events with the need of emergent cardiovascular surgery and neurologic death in hospital. At 6-month follow-up, 1 patient had an ischemic stroke. Implantation and treatment success was met in 96% and 97% of cases. On transesophageal echocardiography

only 14 patients (13%) showed mild to moderate leaks around the device. In addition, no mobile thrombi or impairment of mitral valve and pulmonary vein function was found. Procedure-related serious adverse events occurred in a total of 9 patients. Two patients had pericardial effusion and another 2 patients had cardiac tamponade. One patient had left-sided hemothorax and 1 patient developed deep vein thrombosis. Two strokes were observed during the follow-up, 1 at day 173 and another at day 215 after PLAATO implantation. Hence, the observed annual stroke rate was 2.2%.

The study group concluded that PLAATO may be performed successfully at an acceptable risk and requested further larger studies.

COMPLICATIONS AND PROBLEMS

Although the feasibility of percutaneous LAA occlusion was shown, important issues remained. Prevention of thromboembolism and stroke is a prophylactic step. Therefore, even a low risk of serious adverse events is not acceptable during the implantation procedure. Pericardial effusion is a potential life-threatening problem and requires immediate action. Hence, patient selection and risk assessment for stroke are of particular importance. Because the study mainly enrolled patients who were contraindicated to oral anticoagulants, the performance of the device was not compared with patients eligible for oral anticoagulants. Residual leaks may cause thrombus formation. Furthermore, the role of antiplatelet therapy was not systematically investigated. Nevertheless, at least in a large cohort of patients, the combined use of acetylic acid and clopidogrel was associated with a very low rate of thrombus formation of the device. The need and duration of dual antiplatelet therapy, however, were not addressed. The physiologic effects of LAA occlusion were not investigated and investigators encouraged formal investigation of the physiologic effects after PLAATO.[17,18] Unfortunately, larger studies could not be founded by the company and eventually the device was removed from the market in 2005.

POSTMORTEM ANALYSIS IN HUMANS

In 2005, the authors reported on a patient who died 1 year after the implantation of the device from a perimyocarditis.[19] The LAA was completely occluded by the device and a complete neointima had developed over the device. Leaks were not found. The device was partly protruding into the cavity of the left atrium. Due its ball shape, more than two-thirds of the device was adjacent to the walls of the LAA. Behind the device, the LAA cavity contained an organized thrombus, indicating secondary distal thrombosis after implantation of the device.

In contrast to these findings, Park and colleagues[20] did not find neo-endothelialization of the atrial surface of a PLAATO device 2.5 years after successful implantation in a postmortem case. This finding raises concerns to the individual healing process after implantation of LAA occlusion devices.[20]

LONG-TERM FOLLOW-UP

The 5-year results of the PLAATO study were reported separately by a North American working group and a European working group. Block and colleagues[21] reported in 2009 for the first group. They followed 64 patients for an average of 3.8 years. A total of 18 major adverse events were reported: 7 deaths, 5 major strokes, 3 minor strokes, 1 cardiac tamponade requiring surgery, 1 probable cerebral hemorrhage/death, and 1 myocardial infarction. The estimated annual stroke risk was 6.6%, whereas the observed stroke rate was only 3.8%.

The European PLAATO study group reported on 180 patients with nonrheumatic atrial fibrillation and contraindications to OAC. In the study group, the expected annual stroke rate was also 6.6%. The observed rate, however, was only 2.3%. In 1 patient, the device chosen was too small and embolized in the aorta, where the device was snared and retrieved.[22]

Between September 2001 and 2005, the authors implanted the PLAATO device in 40 patients with atrial fibrillation.[23] The mean age was 71.3 years $\pm$ 8.2 years. The average CHA_2DS_2 VASc (Score for atrial fibrillation stroke risk) score was 4.6 $\pm$ 1.7. Patients were followed up to 15 years after implantation; 1 patient had a major stroke during follow-up, resulting in an annual stroke rate of 0.25%, and 8 patients had a transesophageal echocardiographic follow-up after 10 years. In all cases, the device was in typical position and no thrombi were found on the surface of the device.

ALTERNATIVE TECHNOLOGIES

In 2003, Meier and colleagues[24] reported on transcatheter LAA occlusion with the Amplatzer (AGA Medical Corporation, Plymouth, MN) atrial septal defect device in 16 patients. The left disc of the device was deployed within the LAA,

whereas the right part of the device was released at the entrance of the appendage "like the pacifier plate outside a baby's mouth." The position of the device was confirmed both by contrast injection and intracardiac echocardiography. Device embolization occurred in 1 patient with an atrial septal defect. The patient underwent elective surgical device removal. Echocardiographic follow-up showed complete occlusion of the LAA without thrombus formation on the atrial surface of the device. One year after successful implantation of the PLAATO device the first WATCHMAN device (Atritec Inc, Plymouth, MN) was implanted. Detailed information on the history of both implantation techniques are found in this issue.

SUMMARY

Percutaneous LAA occlusion was introduced as an alternative method for prevention of thromboembolism in patients with nonvalvular atrial fibrillation after extensive animal work in 2001. The first device was named PLAATO (no longer sold or produced) and the device was invented by Michael Lesh, MD.

REFERENCES

1. Kirchhoff P, Benussi S, Kotecha D, et al. 2016 ESC Guidelines for the management of atrial fibrillation. Eur Heart J 2016;37:2893–962.
2. Calenda B, Fuster V, Halperin J, et al. Stroke risk assessment in atrial fibrillation: risk factors and marker of atrial myopathy. Nat Rev Cardiol 2016; 13:549–59.
3. Olesen J, Lip G, Hansen M, et al. Validation of risk stratification schemes for predicting stroke and thromboembolism in patients with atrial fibrillation: nationwide cohort study. BMJ 2011;342:1–9.
4. Mügge A, Kühn H, Nikutta P, et al. Assessment of left atrial appendage function by biplane transesophageal echocardiography in patients with nonrheumatic atrial fibrillation: identification of a subgroup of patients at increased embolic risk. J Am Coll Cardiol 1994;23:599–607.
5. Fatkin D, Kelly RP, Fenely MP. Relations between left atrial appendage blood flow velocity, spontaneous echocardiographic contrast and thromboembolic risk in vivo. J Am Coll Cardiol 1994;23:961–9.
6. Stroke Prevention in Atrial Fibrillation Investigators. Adjusted-dose warfarin versus low-intensity, fixed dose warfarin plus aspirin for high-risk patients with atrial fibrillation: Stroke Prevention in Atrial Fibrillation III randomized clinical trial. Lancet 1996;348:633–8.
7. Lip G, Laroche C, Dan G, et al. 'Real-World' antithrombotic treatment in atrial fibrillation: the EORP-AF Pilot survey. Am J Med 2014;127:519–29.

8. Sievert H, Lesh MD, Trepels T, et al. Percutaneous left atrial appendage transcatheter occlusion to prevent stroke in high-risk patients with atrial fibrillation: early clinical experiences. Circulation 2002; 105:1887–9.

9. Aschenberg W, Schlüter M, Kremer P, et al. Transesophageal two-dimesional echocardiography for the detection of left atrial appendage thrombus. J Am Coll Cardiol 1986;7:163–6.

10. Pandian NG, Hsu TL, Schwartz SL, et al. Multiplane transesophageal echocardiography. Imaging planes, echocardiographic anatomy, and clinical experience with a prototype phased array OmniPlane probe. Echocardiography 1992;9:649–66.

11. Flachskampf F, Hoffmann R, Verlande M, et al. Initial experience with a multiplane transesophageal echotransducer: assessment of diagnostic potential. Eur Heart J 1992;13:1201–6.

12. Omran H, Jung W, Rabahieh R, et al. Left atrial chamber and appendage function after internal atrial defibrillation: a prospective and serial transesophageal echocardiographic study. J Am Coll Cardiol 1997;29(1):131–8.

13. US patent number 6,152,144. Issued 2000. Appriva Medical, Inc.

14. Nakai T, Lesh MD, Gerstenfeld EP, et al. Percutaneous left atrial appendage occlusion (PLAATO) for preventing cardioembolism: first experience in canine model. Circulation 2002;105(18):2217–22.

15. Nakai T, Lesh M, Ostermayer S, et al. An endovascular approach to cardioembolic stroke prevention in atrial fibrillation patients. Pacing Clin Electrophysiol 2003;26(7 Pt 2):1604–6.

16. Ostermayer SH, Reisman M, Kramer PH, et al. Percutaneous left atrial appendage transcatheter occlusion (PLAATO system) to prevent stroke in high-risk patients with non-rheumatic atrial fibrillation: results from the international multi-center feasibility trials. J Am Coll Cardiol 2005;46(1):9–14.

17. Schneider B, Finsterer J, Stöllberger C. Effects of percutaneous left atrial appendage transcatheter occlusion (PLAATO) on left atrial structure and function. J Am Coll Cardiol 2005;45(4):634–5 [author reply: 635].

18. Ostermayer S, Reschke M, Billinger K, et al. Percutaneous closure of the left atrial appendage. J Interv Cardiol 2003;16(6):553–6.

19. Omran H, Schmidt H, Hardung D, et al. Post mortem analysis of a left atrial appendage occlusion device (PLAATO) in a patient with permanent atrial fibrillation. J Interv Card Electrophysiol 2005;14(1): 17–20.

20. Park JW, Gerk U, Franke RP, et al. Post-mortem analysis of a left atrial appendage occlusion system (PLAATO) in a patient with permanent atrial fibrillation. Cardiology 2009;112:205–8.

21. Block PC, Burstein S, Casale PN, et al. Percutaneous left atrial appendage occlusion for patients in atrial fibrillation suboptimal for warfarin therapy: 5-year results of the PLAATO (Percutaneous Left Atrial Appendage Transcatheter Occlusion) Study. JACC Cardiovasc Interv 2009; 2(7):594–600.

22. Bayard YL, Omran H, Neuzil P, et al. PLAATO (Percutaneous Left Atrial Appendage Transcatheter Occlusion) for prevention of cardioembolic stroke in non-anticoagulation eligible atrial fibrillation patients: results from the European PLAATO study. EuroIntervention 2010;6:220–6.

23. Omran H, Hardung D, Schmidt H, et al. Mechanical occlusion of the left atrial appendage. J Cardiovasc Electrophysiol 2003;14(9 Suppl): S56–9.

24. Meier B, Palacios I, Windecker S, et al. Transcatheter left atrial appendage occlusion with amplatzer devices to obviate anticoagulation in patients with atrial fibrillation. Catheter Cardiovasc Interv 2003; 60:417–22.

A History of Left Atrial Appendage Occlusion

David R. Holmes Jr, MD[a],*, Robert S. Schwartz, MD[b], George G. Latus, BSBME[c], Robert A. Van Tassel, MD[d]

KEYWORDS

- Left atrial appendage • Atrial fibrillation • Watchman ablation strategy • Antiembolic therapy

---

KEY POINTS

- A new era in antiembolic therapy has been initiated by the growing numbers of device-based therapies to locally and mechanically isolate and occlude the left atrial appendage (LAA).
- Other benefits are being further evaluated, such as the possibility of achieving a striking reduction in mortality with device implantation and avoidance of long-term anticoagulation that was documented in the Watchman limbs of the randomized controlled trials.
- Many other questions remain, such as whether there is a device-specific outcome effect or whether it is a class effect.
- It is now scientifically proven that the LAA using the Watchman ablation strategy can successfully reduce cardioembolic stroke, with comparable or fewer adverse effects by device technology than obtained by long-term anticoagulation with its attendant bleeding risks.
- This information is the latest in the paradigm of local mechanical therapy replacing systemic pharmacology treatments for the prevention of stroke in patients with nonvalvular atrial fibrillation.

Atrial fibrillation and the left atrial appendage (LAA) have been long associated with embolic stroke, and this association is now a proven causal relationship.[1-3] Atrial fibrillation has strong age-dependent prevalence as does stroke, and both are associated with serious morbidity and mortality. Madden reported 2 cases in 1949 where "resection of the left auricular appendix was performed in the human being as prophylaxis for recurring arterial thrombi."[4] Both patients (a 32-year-old woman and a 52-year-old man) had histories of rheumatic heart disease, and thrombi were found in the LAA of each at surgery.

Since then multiple surgical- and more recently catheter-based approaches to LAA

ablation have been developed, tested, approved, and clinically applied. Efficacy data from these novel device-based strategies include observational studies, registries, and randomized clinical trials.[5-19]

The LAA is an enigmatic anatomic structure whose function has only recently been understood. It forms during the fourth week of embryonic development, and is exquisitely fragile (Fig. 1), with paper-thin walls interspersed with numerous pectinate muscles. Johnson[20] called the LAA "the most lethal human attachment" because of its propensity to tear. The shape is complex, and frequently multi-lobed. It has been characterized in specific morphologies by computed tomography (CT)

---

[a] Department of Cardiovascular Diseases, Mayo Clinic College of Medicine, Mayo Clinic, 200 First Street SW, Rochester, MN 55905, USA; [b] Advanced Imaging Research, Minneapolis Heart Institute, 920 E. 28th Street, Minneapolis, MN 55407, USA; [c] Boston Scientific, 4100 Hamline Avenue N, St Paul, MN 55112, USA; [d] Minneapolis Heart Institute Foundation, 800 E. 28th Street, Minneapolis, MN 55407, USA
* Corresponding author.
E-mail address: holmes.david@mayo.edu

Intervent Cardiol Clin 7 (2018) 143–150
https://doi.org/10.1016/j.iccl.2017.12.005
2211-7458/18/© 2017 Elsevier Inc. All rights reserved.

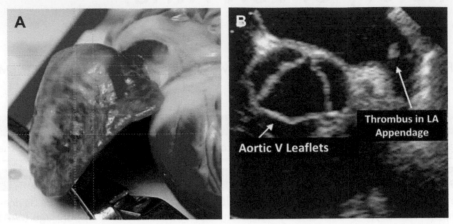

Fig. 1. (A) The LAA, external view. The bellows-like shape is mechanistically optimized as an efficient left atrial pressure sensor. ANP synthesis and secretion from within the LAA myocardium is likely regulated by LA pressure to optimize myocardial filling. (B) TEE image showing thrombus in the LAA from a patient with chronic Atrial fibrillation.

imagining-windsock, chicken wing, cactus, and cauliflower. This classification scheme is helpful in preprocedural planning to increase success and to reduce complication risk.

The LAA myocardium is rich in both ANP and BNP, and has a bellows-like shape, making it a sensitive LA pressure transducer and regulator of left ventricular end-diastolic pressure (LVEDP). It thus serves key endocrine functions relating to body fluid and electrolyte management. The clinical effects of these functions in older patients with multiple comorbidities and chronic persistent AF are neither well understood nor quantitated.[21]

Blackshear and Odell[22] provided seminal observations with profound implications for LAA relevance to cardioembolic stroke in atrial fibrillation. They found the LAA was a thrombus source in 90% of all cardioembolic events. This contrasts with valvular AF patients (principally mitral valve stenosis) where only 57% of thrombi originated in LAA, with the remainder arising from the left atrium itself. This finding provided key clinical implications for patient selection in LAA ablation, restricting its application only to those patients with nonvalvular atrial fibrillation (NVAF).

These data were published on the background of anticoagulation (principally warfarin) as the standard of care for long-term preventive strategies for stroke prophylaxis. Warfarin simultaneously was shown effective against stroke, but had substantive clinical inconvenience including the need for monitoring, drug-drug interactions, genetic variability in dose response, and sometimes serious bleeding. Warfarin

therapy moreover developed a long list of contraindications, due especially to its potential for hemorrhage, highest in the elderly population who concurrently have the highest atrial fibrillation prevalence and need for anticoagulant-based stroke prevention.[23]

These issues led to newer anticoagulants (novel oral anticoagulants [NOACs] or direct oral anticoagulants [DOACs]), which were potentially safer and more convenient.[24,25] They did not, however, alleviate relative and absolute contraindications to anticoagulant therapy. Other concerns included a lack of widely available antidotes to bleeding, a need to adjust dose in patients with renal disease, a twice daily dosing regimen, cost, and noncompliance. These considerations are significant problems as shown in a recent administrative data base of 64,661 patients at a median follow-up of 1.1 years.[26] These data show that only approximately 50% of patients at stroke risk in this setting were taking appropriate anticoagulants.

Recognition of the LAA as a key component in cardioembolic events and significant drawbacks to medical (anticoagulant) therapy raised the question of whether device-based interventional, local, and specific occlusive therapy could be a viable alternative.

The Watchman was an early device to successfully occlude the LAA (Fig. 2). The very name alludes to the classic but never-delivered speech by President John Fitzgerald Kennedy in Dallas, Texas, on November 22, 1963, in which he was to deliver the classic words about "watchman on the walls." This

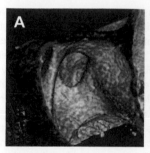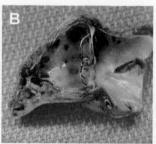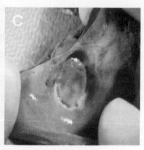

Fig. 2. (A) The LAA orifice as visualized from the atrial septum. VRT image from a patient in sinus rhythm. (B) Early prototype Watchman device in a canine LAA. Note endocardium seals the atrial interface, and connects with the left atrial rim, making a complete seal. (C) LAA ablation in a canine by the Watchman device. Complete seal is again shown, utilizing biocompatible polymer covering. Identical results occur in humans.

biblical concept could be amended to apply to devices used for stroke prevention. The Watchman device was conceived in times of coronary artery stenting, and designed analogously to the stent paradigm; if coronary stents could keep biologic structures patent, stent-like design modifications (balloon-expandable or self-expanding) could be adapted to apply to a design that could occlude structures such as the LAA.

Successful LAA occlusion by the Watchman in preclinical studies resulted in 2 US Food and Drug Administration (FDA) randomized clinical trials and 2 continued access registries during FDA review and eventual device approval with expected postapproval registries and continued data collection.[17-19] Other devices developed in the same era included the PLAATO device.[8,9] The first human implants of the PLAATO device occurred in August 2001, approximately 1 year prior to the first human Watchman implants. The Watchman went through multiple design iterations including enhanced fixation anchors and a biocompatible, semipermeable polymer surface membrane that provided a scaffold for endocardial sealing after healing (see Fig. 2) within a short timeframe of an estimated 6 to 12 weeks after implant based on prior animal research. The device was conceived and developed by interventional cardiologists working with engineers in a medical device startup company (Atritech, Plymouth Minnesota, 2000) having extensive medical device engineering and clinical experience.

Much of the early work in device design was based bench testing. From an intellectual property standpoint of bench testing and differentiating device design, it was decided to pursue an open-end distal design as well as a semipermeable positron emission tomography (PET) fabric covering rather than a closed-end

design and PTFE covering. These features proved to be important enhancements that allowed the Watchman to accommodate a greater range of LAA anatomies and also promote faster and more complete tissue healing with device incorporation into the endocardium.

Early devices were awkward. Subsequent iterations influenced by bench and preclinical testing provided greatly improved performance and biologic/medical results. An important consideration was the possibility of thrombus formation on the polymer membrane surface early after implant. An obvious approach was brief anticoagulation (warfarin) after implantation. Key questions were how long and how much, although without data available for guidance. Preclinical study showed that warfarin therapy for 6 weeks allowed intimal device covering and excellent sealing.[27] This favorable preclinical assessment was never subjected to rigorous testing, although it was clinically accepted. Viewed from a perspective 10 to 15 years later, relevant data remain unavailable.

Working closely with the FDA, Atritech began human clinical studies in 2002. Early clinical experience formed the basis for subsequent clinical studies that resulted in 2 successful randomized clinical trials[18,19] with major implications for instructions for use. The concept of trial design and implementation was daunting, so much so that the competing PLAATO device was abandoned after the regulatory hurdles and costs of starting the randomized clinical trial were not felt to be economically feasible.

During this time the implant procedure evolved rapidly with a steep early learning curve. Eventual implant methods developed into a host of approaches such as careful consideration of patient anatomy, greater emphasis on patient screening, increased diligence and vigilance with catheter manipulation into the LAA, and eliminating potential air embolism sources during catheter exchanges. These all resulted in the improved outcomes seen in the subsequent family of trials and registries.

During early Watchman development, the NOAC oral anticoagulants were approved and studied concomitantly with the Watchman for use in NVAF. The first NOAC candidate studied extensively with the hope of FDA approval was EXANTA. This, however, was never approved due principally to liver toxicity. Other NOAC studies began in earnest with approval of Dabigatran beginning in October 2010. Speculation about clinical safety, efficacy, and final use of these drugs complicated questions of device-based LAA ablation therapy. Such questions also included market penetration and size, and patient population.

In lengthy regulatory conversations with the FDA, multiple issues were raised and addressed (Box 1). These interactions had profound implications for device design and testing methods, and were applied later to other LAA devices. The optimal patient population was a crucial decision and defaulted to those patients felt to be unable to take long-term anticoagulation. Such patients constituted a sizable unmet clinical need. Yet the complex issues of relative versus absolute contraindications were poorly defined. Those issues remain current today with devices and patient selection. Related and unanswered questions concern the need for short-term anticoagulation to enhance neo-endocardial tissue covering to prevent device-associated thrombosis. This question bears on proper anticoagulant dosing and duration. Preclinical studies did not rigorously examine anticoagulation, defaulting to 6 weeks based on early animal data for endocardial covering.

Six weeks became the patient standard, who for trial participation were required to take this short-term anticoagulation for 6 weeks. These data were available during the regulatory approval submission. Early regulatory discussions centered around the large unmet clinical need in patients in whom anticoagulants were felt to be contraindicated even for a short time. Efforts to engage the sponsor to either amend the protocol or begin a new parallel trial in patients who were not candidates for anticoagulation were unsuccessful for several reasons. These included the challenge of a control population that would receive no therapy as well as the smaller population considered available in order to complete the PROTECT AF study enrollment in a timely fashion. In the scientific arena of a randomized Watchman clinical trial with no anticoagulation, what would the control group look like? If patients were unable to take any anticoagulation, how would the control group be treated? Answers ranged from nothing to aspirin (poor choice) or clopidogrel (no data). Would such a control group be acceptable to the multiplicity of IRBs involved in a pivotal trial? These considerations presaged the ASAP-TOO trial,[28] which has now been initiated 15 years later. This specific trial of LAA closure in patients in whom anticoagulation is contraindicated is of major clinical interest to the clinical community and regulatory agencies as it is a large unmet clinical need.

There were other issues, principally what specific endpoints would be used and how to adjudicate them. There were no ideal answers for all questions.

Device-based site-specific therapy could theoretically only prevent strokes from the LAA (eg, ischemic stroke), but not from other anatomic and physiologic sources that might be prevented by oral anticoagulation. Thus began the anticoagulation debate of systemic versus the local protection from stroke that LAA closure potentially offered. Much early clinical trial discussion centered around whether only ischemic strokes should be an endpoint or whether all strokes would be a better choice. Hemorrhagic stroke inclusion was another question debated intensively. Hemorrhagic strokes would hypothetically occur only with anticoagulant therapy, raising a question whether they should be a primary endpoint. A final clinical trial concern was mortality, either cerebrovascular or all-cause. As part of this discussion, endpoints could be judged using either frequentist or Bayesian models of superiority versus noninferiority. If noninferiority was chosen, what would

---

Box 1
Design issues

Patient population – anticoagulant contraindicated or not?

Trial endpoints – all stroke versus ischemic stroke, composite or single

Selection criteria

Periprocedural meds

Site selection

Postprocedural testing

Superiority versus noninferiority – frequentist versus Bayesian

be the boundary of significance for the end-points? In a field with a new type or class of device, never tested in a randomized trial, the arbitrary selection of a specific boundary has great implications but is hard to identify in the absence of data.

Periprocedural medication selection was also important. FDA guidance suggested warfarin for 6 weeks. The trials and subsequent instructions for use thus include 6 weeks of warfarin. In those early times, NOACs were unavailable for incorporation into trials, and were not used. Therefore, detailed well-controlled randomized scientific study of NOACs in combination with LAA closure devices or as alternative approaches for stroke prevention is not available. Even today, such information is only available anecdotally from either single or multicenter registries. Other related questions included what follow-up testing would be required such as the need for TEE, and if so, what was the sequence and need for rigorous detailed neurologic testing.

A final question with increasing importance is that of residual leaks. In the surgical LAA closure or ablation literature, residual leaks have been associated with recurrent thromboembolic events. Residual leaks have now been studied for LAA closure with devices. The prevalence is poorly defined, but early data suggest that a residual leak less than 5 mm is not associated with increased stroke and thromboembolism hazard.[29] This definition of residual leak was arbitrary based on information from devices used for PFO and ASD closures. Work continues to quantify the occurrence of leaks as well as approaches to minimize them.

The journey from first patient enrollment with the Watchman device began with enrollment in a pilot study initiated at Mayo Clinic in October 2003. This feasibility study was successful and led to the multicenter randomized PROTECT AF[18] clinical trial. Mayo Clinic enrolled their first PROTECT AF patient on October 31, 2006,

which subsequently gave rise to a second randomized trial PREVAIL,[19] with 2 accompanying clinical registries for final FDA approval March 13, 2015, and then to CMS approval February 8, 2016. This journey included 2406 patients followed in aggregate at the time of the last FDA panel meeting, totaling 5931 patient-years. Three FDA panel meetings were held on the Watchman device for the same patient indication groups,[30] an unprecedented record of dubious distinction where all 3 FDA panels were in fact positive, and at an incremental cost in excess of more than $200,000,000. The 3 FDA panel meetings highlighted the previously discussed issues of patient selection, trial design, endpoints used, and statistical analysis. As can be seen, the results of each FDA panel varied (Table 1). The first panel (April 24, 2009) included a vote for approval (7–5). Despite this successful vote, a nonapprovable letter was received directing the company to obtain more data with a second randomized controlled trial (PREVAIL) to include higher-risk patients and an accompanying registry. PREVAIL began November 1, 2010, and culminated in a second FDA panel approval (December 2013). By this time, FDA panel voting procedures changed and included votes on safety, efficacy and positive benefit/risk profile. Votes in this panel were consistent at 13 to 1, but approval was again deferred, because unexpectedly, the second randomized controlled trial had not met all 3 prespecified endpoints. Multiple reasons were considered as plausible and included better than expected control group results, and concerns about ischemic versus hemorrhagic stroke as relevant study endpoints. Continued evaluation of the growing duration of follow-up data available resulted in a third and final panel, held October 8, 2014 with unanimously favorable results (12–0) for safety, 6 to 7 for efficacy (the FDA panel chair had voted because of a tie vote, and 6–5 for positive benefit/risk profile). FDA approval followed on March 13, 2015, with the current IFU (Box 2).[31] After

Table 1			
US Food and Drug Administration circulatory panel voting			
	2009 Panel 4/23/09	**2013 Panel 12/11/13**	**2014 Panel 10/8/14**
For approval	7–5	N/A	N/A
Safety	N/A	13–1	12–0
Efficacy	N/A	13–1	6–7 (chair voted to break tie)
Positive benefit/risk Profile	N/A	13–1	6–5 (one abstain)

Box 2
March 2015 Watchman instructions for use

The Watchman device is indicated to reduce the risk of thromboembolism from the left atrial appendage in patients with nonvalvular atrial fibrillation who:

- Are at increased risk for stroke and systemic embolism based on CHADS$_2$ or CHA$_2$DS$_2$-VASc scores and are recommended for anticoagulation therapy;
- Are deemed by their physicians to be suitable for warfarin
- Have an appropriate rationale to seek a nonpharmacologic alternative to warfarin, taking into account the safety and effectiveness of the device compared with warfarin

Box 3
US reimbursement status CMS national coverage decision (February 8, 2016)

Criteria for coverage:

- CHADS$_2$ score ≥ 2 or CHA$_2$DS$_2$-VASc score ≥ 3
- A formal shared decision making interaction with an independent noninterventional physician using an evidence-based decision tool on oral anticoagulation in patients with NVAF
- Suitable for short-term warfarin but deemed unable to take long-term oral anticoagulation

FDA approval, additional processes included CMS evaluation included a robust and lengthy comment period. This culminated in CMS reimbursement approval on February 8, 2016.[32] This approval, however, came with specific caveats (Box 3), including an obligatory enrollment of all patients after approval in a national registry. The national coverage determination mandated a more formal shared decision making process as a requirement for approval.[33] This requirement has been difficult to interpret and implement for multiple reasons. The requirement for reimbursement involving the shared decision making process may have important implications for all new technology going forward if that model is chosen.

From October 2006 to FDA approval, the Watchman device remained unchanged in terms of frame shape and overall device length, materials used, and fixation method. During this time, however, robust global application of the Watchman device used in the initial randomized controlled trials began, although with different patient selection criteria. This process resulted in multiple registries, which have highlighted current practice and focus on issues of anticoagulation need after the procedure. In current global practice, Watchman is used in patients at high stroke risk, many of whom are not treated with anticoagulation. This expanding data set with large international registries such as EWOLUTION[10] potentially answers the question of need for anticoagulation before ASAP-TOO[28] finishes enrollment. The data from these registries have informed the IFU for Watchman placement (Table 2).

Table 2
Watchman indications for use – comparison of US and European Union

US Indication	European Union Indication
The Watchman device is indicated to reduce the risk of thromboembolism from the left atrial appendage in patients with nonvalvular atrial fibrillation who: • Are at increased risk for stroke and systemic embolism based on CHADS$_2$ or CHA$_2$DS$_2$-VASc scores and are recommended for anticoagulation therapy • Are deemed by their physicians to be suitable for warfarin; and • Have an appropriate rationale to seek a nonpharmacologic alternative to warfarin, taking into account the safety and effectiveness of the device compared with warfarin	The Watchman LAA closure technology is intended to prevent thrombus embolization from the LAA and reduce the risk of life-threatening bleeding events in patients with nonvalvular atrial fibrillation who are eligible for anticoagulation therapy or who have a contraindication to anticoagulation therapy

SUMMARY

A new era in antiembolic therapy has been initiated by the growing numbers of device-based therapies to locally and mechanically isolate and occlude the LAA. Early concerns surrounding eliminating this enigmatic structure, some catastrophic, have not proven true. Other benefits are being further evaluated, such as the possibility of achieving a striking reduction in mortality with device implantation and avoidance of long-term anticoagulation that was documented in the Watchman limbs of the randomized controlled trials. Many other questions remain, such as whether there is a device-specific outcome effect or whether it is a class effect. Other questions include other devices, what head-to-head studies will show, and the impact of residual leak. It is now scientifically proven that the LAA using the Watchman ablation strategy can successfully reduce cardioembolic stroke, with comparable or fewer side effects by device technology than obtained by long-term anticoagulation with its attendant bleeding risks. This information is the latest in the paradigm of local mechanical therapy replacing systemic pharmacology treatments for the prevention of stroke in patients with NVAF.

REFERENCES

1. Wolf PA, Abbott RD, Kannel WB. Atrial fibrillation as an independent risk factor for stroke: the Framingham Study. Stroke 1991;22:983–8.
2. Lip GYH, Brechin CM, Lane DA. The global burden of atrial fibrillation and stroke: a systematic review of the epidemiology of atrial fibrillation in regions outside North American and Europe. Chest 2012; 142:1489–98.
3. Schnabel RB, Yin X, Gona P, et al. 50 year trends in atrial fibrillation prevalence, incidence, risk factors, and mortality in the Framingham Heart Study; a cohort study. Lancet 2015;386:154–62.
4. Madden JL. Resection of the left auricular appendix; a prophylaxis for recurrent arterial emboli. J Am Med Assoc 1949;140:769–72.
5. Holmes DR, Reddy VY. Left atrial appendage and closure: who, when and how. Circ Cardiovasc Interv 2016;9(5):e002942.
6. Meier B, Blaauw Y, Khattab AA, et al. EHRA/EAPCI expert consensus statement on catheter-based left atrial appendage occlusion. EuroIntervention 2015; 10:1109–25.
7. Lakkireddy D, Afzal MR, Lee RJ, et al. Short and long-term outcomes of percutaneous left atrial appendage suture ligation: results from a US multicenter evaluation. Heart Rhythm 2016;13:1030–6.
8. Ostermayer SH, Reisman M, Kramer PH, et al. Percutaneous left atrial appendage transcatheter occlusion (PLAATO system) to prevent stroke in high-risk patients with non-rheumatic atrial fibrillation: results from the international multi-center feasibility trials. J Am Coll Cardiol 2005;46:9–14.
9. Bayard YL, Omran H, Neuzil P, et al. PLAATO (percutaneous left atrial appendage transcatheter occlusion) for prevention of cardioembolic stroke in non-anticoagulation eligible atrial fibrillation patients: results from the European PLAATO study. EuroIntervention 2010;6:220–6.
10. Boersma LV, Schmidt B, Betts TR, et al. Implant success and safety of left atrial appendage closure with the WATCHMAN device: peri-procedural outcomes from the EWOLUTION registry. Eur Heart J 2016;37:2465–71.
11. Cox JL. Mechanical closure of the left atrial appendage: is it time to be more aggressive? J Thorac Cardiovasc Surg 2013;146:1018–27.
12. Healey JS, Crystal E, Lamy A, et al. Left atrial appendage occlusion study (LAAOS): results of a randomized controlled pilot study of left atrial appendage occlusion during coronary bypass surgery in patients at risk for stroke. Am Heart J 2005;150:288–93.
13. Emmert MY, Puippe G, Baumuller S, et al. Safe, effective and durable epicardial left atrial appendage clip occlusion in patients with atrial fibrillation undergoing cardiac surgery: first long-term results form a prospective device trial. Eur J Cardiothorac Surg 2014;45:126–31.
14. Tzikas A, Shakir S, Gafoor S, et al. Left atrial appendage occlusion for stroke prevention in atrial fibrillation: multicenter experience with the AMPLATZER cardiac plug. EuroIntervention 2016; 11:1170–9.
15. Reddy VY, Mobius-Winkler S, Miller MA, et al. Left atrial appendage closure with the Watchman device in patients with a contraindication for oral anticoagulation: the ASAP study (ASA plavix feasibility study with watchman left atrial appendage closure technology). J Am Coll Cardiol 2013;61:2551–6.
16. Reddy VY, Gibson DN, Kar S, et al. Post-approval U.S. experience with left atrial appendage closure for stroke prevention in atrial fibrillation. J Am Coll Cardiol 2017;69:253–61.
17. Holmes DR, Doshi SK, Kar S, et al. Left atrial appendage closure as an alternative to Warfarin for stroke prevention in atrial fibrillation: a patient-level meta-analysis. J Am Coll Cardiol 2015;65:2614–23.
18. Holmes DR, Reddy VY, Turi ZG, et al. Percutaneous closure of the left atrial appendage versus warfarin therapy for prevention of stroke in patients with atrial fibrillation: a randomized non-inferiority trial. Lancet 2009;374:534–42.

19. Holmes DR, Kar S, Price MJ, et al. Prospective randomized evaluation of the Watchman left atrial appendage closure device in patients with atrial fibrillation versus long-term warfarin therapy: the PREVAIL trial. J Am Coll Cardiol 2014;64:1–12.

20. Johnson WD, Ganjoo AK, Stone CD, et al. The left atrial appendage: our most lethal human attachment! Surgical implications. Eur J Cardiothorac Surg 2000;17:718–22.

21. Majunke N, Sandri M, Adams V, et al. Atrial and brain natriuretic peptide secretion after percutaneous closure of the left atrial appendage with the Watchman device. J Invasive Cardiol 2015;27:448–52.

22. Blackshear JL, Odell JA. Appendage obliteration to reduce stroke in cardiac surgical patients with atrial fibrillation. Ann Thorac Surg 1996;61:755–9.

23. Lip G, Lip GYH, Freedman B, et al. Stroke prevention in atrial fibrillation: past, present and future. Comparing the guidelines and practical decision-making. Thromb Haemost 2017;117:1230–9.

24. Heidbuchel H, Verhamme P, Alings M, et al. Updated European Heart Rhythm Association practical guide on the use of non-vitamin-K antagonist anticoagulants in patients with non-valvular atrial fibrillation: executive summary. Eur Heart J 2017;38(27):2137–49.

25. Ruff CT, Giugliano RP, Braunwald E, et al. Comparison of the efficacy and safety of new oral anticoagulants with warfarin in patients with atrial fibrillation: a meta-analysis of randomized trials. Lancet 2014;383:955–62.

26. Yao X, Abraham NS, Alexander G, et al. Effect of adherence to oral anticoagulants on risk of stroke and major bleeding among patients with atrial fibrillation. J Am Heart Assoc 2016;5(2) [pii:e003074].

27. Schwartz RS, Holmes DR, Van Tassel RA, et al. Left atrial appendage obliteration: mechanisms of healing and intracardiac integration. JACC Cardiovasc Interv 2010;3:870–7.

28. Holmes DR, Reddy VY, Buchbinder M, et al. The assessment of the Watchman device in patients unsuitable for oral anticoagulation (ASAP-TOO) trial. Am Heart J 2017;189:68–74.

29. Viles-Gonzalez JF, Kar S, Douglas P, et al. The clinical impact of incomplete left atrial appendage closure with the Watchman device in patients with atrial fibrillation. J Am Coll Cardiol 2012;59:923–9. Available at: http://www.ncbi.nlm.nih.gov/pubmed/22381428. Accessed June 29, 2017.

30. Waksman R, Pendyala LK. Overview of the Food and Drug Administration circulatory system devices panel meetings on Watchman left atrial appendage closure therapy. Am J Cardiol 2015;115:378–84.

31. Watchman LAA. Closure technology – P130013. 2016. Available at: https://www.fda.gov/MedicalDevices/ProductsandMedicalProcedures/DeviceApprovalsandClearances/Recently-ApprovedDevices/ucm440621.htm. Accessed June 29, 2017.

32. Decision memo for percutaneous left atrial appendage (LAA) closure therapy (CAG-00445N). Available at: https://www.cms.gov/medicare-coverage-database/details/nca-decision-memo.aspx?NCAId=281. Accessed June 29, 2017.

33. Coylewright M, Holmes DR. Caution regarding government-managed shared decision making for patients with atrial fibrillation. Circulation 2017;135:2211–3.

History of Percutaneous Left Atrial Appendage Occlusion with AMPLATZER Devices

Bernhard Meier, MD[a],*, Wim Stegink, MBA[b],
Apostolos Tzikas, MD, PhD[c]

KEYWORDS

- AMPLATZER devices • Left atrial appendage occlusion • Atrial fibrillation • Stroke prevention

KEY POINTS

- AMPLATZER devices were the first percutaneous occluders used for left atrial appendage closure in the prevention of stroke in patients with atrial fibrillation, except for the no longer available PLAATO device.
- Amulet, the current AMPLATZER device for left atrial appendage occlusion, affords a relatively simple implantation technique requiring fluoroscopy only and no sedation.
- The AMPLATZER technique allows simultaneous closure of atrial septal defects without change of gear.
- Randomized follow-up data with the WATCHMAN device show a mortality benefit versus warfarin treatment. There are supporting AMPLATZER data making this likely a treatment strategy effect.
- Left atrial appendage occlusion should be made accessible for all patients with atrial fibrillation, in the sense of a mechanical vaccination.

INTRODUCTION

Atrial fibrillation is associated with embolic stroke by different mechanisms.[1] The most important one is thrombosis in the left atrial appendage (LAA).[2] The mortality of strokes related to atrial fibrillation is significantly higher than the overall stroke mortality.[3,4] This is because an embolic stroke typically blocks a healthy artery, whereas a stroke based on atherosclerosis may occur after years of an increasing arterial stenosis triggering collateralization of the dependent territory. In contrast to former belief, the stroke risk is higher with persistent or permanent atrial fibrillation than with paroxysmal atrial fibrillation.[5–7] Yet, any type of atrial fibrillation with the exception of the paroxysmal form in an otherwise healthy and young person merits chronic oral anticoagulation[8] or, alternatively, LAA occlusion. The latter reduces the relative stroke risk by about 90%,[2] rendering the remaining risk too small to warrant the complications of oral anticoagulation.

DEVELOPMENT OF LEFT ATRIAL APPENDAGE OCCLUSION WITH AMPLATZER DEVICES

The clinical introduction of percutaneous LAA occlusion by Michael Lesh and Horst Sievert on August 30, 2001,[9] kindled the interest of many an interventional cardiologist. For 50 years, cardiac surgeons had looked into the feasibility and value of LAA occlusion, exclusion, or

[a] Department of Cardiology, University Hospital of Bern, Bern CH-3010, Switzerland; [b] Abbott, Coordination Center, Corporate Village, Da Vinci laan 11, Zaventem 1935, Belgium; [c] AHEPA University Hospital, Interbalkan European Medical Centre, Thessaloniki, Greece
* Corresponding author.
E-mail address: bernhard.meier@insel.ch

Intervent Cardiol Clin 7 (2018) 151–158
https://doi.org/10.1016/j.iccl.2017.12.007
2211-7458/18/© 2017 Elsevier Inc. All rights reserved.

elimination.[10–22] However, the results of these techniques where never properly evaluated and of little interest to interventional cardiologists.

After some initial experiences with the PLAATO device,[9] it occurred that the technique developed by Kurt Amplatz to close atrial septal defects (ASD) was far simpler to handle. When attempting occlusion of an ASD with a double disk AMPLATZER Septal Occluder (ASO), it happened that the left disk was inadvertently opened in the LAA. It then had to be withdrawn with significant force to pull it snug to the interatrial septum before opening the right disk in the right atrium. Hence, ASOs were placed in cadaveric LAAs where they seemed to fit perfectly (Fig. 1). This was the birth of the Bern technique of LAA occlusion, also referred to as the pacifier principle.

Based on an excellent experience of occlusion of ASDs with AMPLATZER devices under fluoroscopic guidance only,[23] echocardiographic guidance was not used (with a few exceptions) when these devices were implanted into the LAA in the first series.[24] Fig. 2 shows the world's first case of catheter-based LAA occlusion with local anesthesia and without echocardiographic guidance. It was performed on June 15, 2002, in Bern, Switzerland. Fig. 3 depicts a modification of the transseptal puncture technique simulating the tenting of the septum primum as seen with transesophageal echocardiography (TEE) by contrast medium injection under fluoroscopy. ASOs 9 mm to 30 mm were used. In one patient with a large ASD, which was planned to be closed at the same time, the 20-mm ASO implanted into the LAA embolized into the left atrium. The patient underwent open-heart surgery to close the LAA and the ASD the following day. Except for one and three of the 16 patients with TEE and intracardiac echocardiography, respectively, fluoroscopic guidance was used exclusively. The cases with echocardiographic guidance were done in centers used to also guide ASD

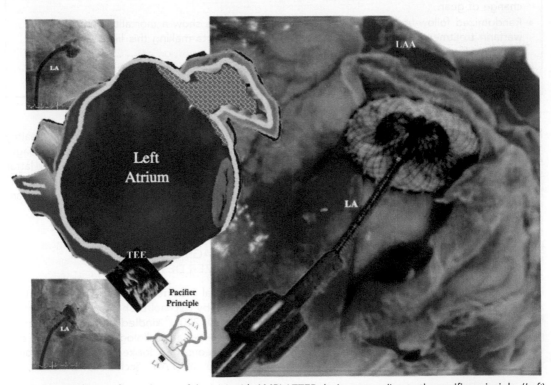

Fig. 1. Bern technique for occlusion of the LAA with AMPLATZER devices according to the pacifier principle. (*Left*) On top the LAA is depicted during contrast filling in a right anterior oblique protection before and, at the bottom, after implantation of an AMPLATZER Cardiac Plug (ACP). The situation is exemplified with a graphic cut through the left atrium (LA) with the distal part of an ACP, or in the example an ASO, compressed in the LAA as an anchor while the proximal disk occludes the LAA orifice. The two center inserts explain the term pacifier principle graphically and by follow-up transesophageal echocardiography (TEE). (*Right*) Occlusion of the LAA in a cadaveric heart with an ASO. The view from the LAA only shows the proximal disk tightly occluding the LAA orifice. The delivery wire is still attached to the female screw of the device. (*Courtesy of* Abbott, Santa Clara, CA; with permission.)

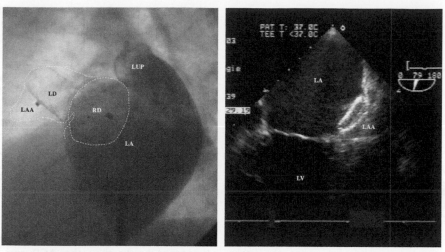

Fig. 2. First in-man catheter-based LAA occlusion under local anesthesia without echocardiographic guidance in a 63-year-old butcher with atrial fibrillation who refused oral anticoagulation for professional reasons. The 30-mm ASO is shown in a left anterior oblique protection on the left and the 1-year-follow-up transesophageal echocardiogram with an excellent result is shown on the right. LA, left atrium; LD, left disk; LUP, left upper pulmonary vein; LV, left ventricle; RD, right disk.

occlusion with TEE. Although this initial series showed excellent long-term results without residual shunts or clots on the device, the technique was no longer pursued because of an acute embolization rate of close to 10% in the first 100 patients.

It was apparent, that the technique needed to be improved on two accounts. First, the mold of the device needed to be adapted to the anatomy of LAAs, which is clearly distinct from the atrial septum. None of the marketed AMPLATZER occluders seemed ideal. Ventricular septal

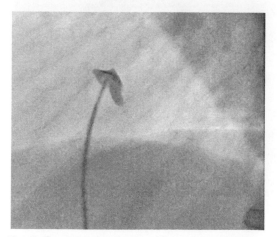

Fig. 3. Transseptal puncture with contrast medium injection through the puncture needle. Dye staining with 0.5 mL of the septum primum in a left anterior oblique projection shows the typical tenting. This identifies a safe place for the transseptal puncture.

defect occluders, patent ductus arteriosus occluders, and patent foramen ovale occluders were tried but their embolization rates were invariably high. Second, the introducer sheath needed a distal curve to allow a deep enough intubation of retroverted LAAs. For the latter, the shape of a right Judkins catheter was suggested but Kurt Amplatz (at the time already retired but still involved and active with improvements and new developments regarding his various cardiac and vascular devices) came up with a 2 × 45°(out of plane) sheath (Fig. 4).

The pacifier principle was forfeited in a prototype single device AMPLATZER LAA occlusion device (Fig. 5). Although it seemed that hooks were essential, Kurt Amplatz was reluctant to include hooks in the design. He recalled bad experiences with hooks when he had initially developed his patent ductus arteriosus occluders. A prototype with retractable hooks was not further pursued.[25] Finally, a double device with a lobe crowned by hooks and a proximal disk reintroducing the pacifier principal was most successful in dog experiments (Fig. 6) and prevailed.

The LAA dedicated device, called AMPLATZER Cardiac Plug (ACP), was clinically first used in Canada[26] and later modified to the Amulet device.[27] It is currently marketed by Abbott after the initial producer AGA Medical had been purchased by St. Jude Medical, which in turn was later acquired by Abbott. It is produced in Plymouth, Minnesota. Table 1 lists the clinically used devices for LAA occlusion that are approved in Europe.

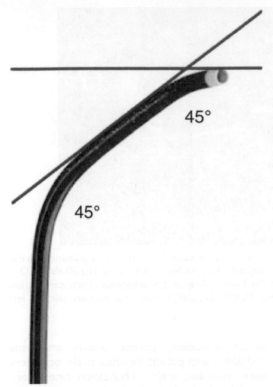

Fig. 4. TorqView 45°/45° sheath for ideal intubation of the various left atrial appendage shapes. The distal 45° bend is out of plane. (*Courtesy of* St. Jude Medical, Inc, Virginia Beach, VA; with permission.)

CLINICAL RESULTS WITH DEDICATED AMPLATZER LEFT ATRIAL APPENDAGE OCCLUSION

The ACP came in sizes of 16 mm, 18 mm, 20 mm, 22 mm, 24 mm, 26 mm, 28 mm, and 30 mm lobe diameter with the proximal disk being 4 mm or 6 mm larger. The Amulet comes in 16 mm, 18 mm, 20 mm, 22 mm, 25 mm, 28 mm, 31 mm, and 34 mm lobe diameters with the disk being 6 mm or 7 mm larger. The lobe depth was 6.5 mm with the ACP and now is 7.5 mm or 10 mm with the Amulet for lobe diameters up to 22 mm or from 25 mm or larger, respectively. For the ACP, sheath sizes of 9F, 10F, and 13F were available. For the Amulet, the sheath sizes are 12F and 14F. The Amulet also has more hooks than the ACP and they are more equally distributed (**Fig. 7**). The Amulet comes preloaded, whereas the ACP had to be loaded into the sheath connector. Lastly, the connector at the left atrial disk side is recessed in the Amulet designed to reduce the risk for thrombus adhesion and the distal end of the pusher cable is redesigned to avoid coiling during advancement, allow easy recapture of the undetached device, and improve flexibility before release.

Dedicated AMPLATZER LAA occlusions showed clear advantages over nondedicated AMPLATZER devices used for LAA occlusion in a

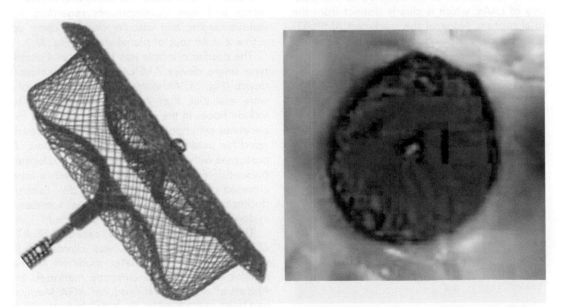

Fig. 5. Prototype nonpacifier AMPLATZER left atrial appendage occlusion device with a proximal disk. (*Left*) Device in profile. (*Right*) View from the left atrium after implantation in a canine left atrial appendage. (*Courtesy of* [*Right panel*] St. Jude Medical, Inc, Virginia Beach, VA; with permission.)

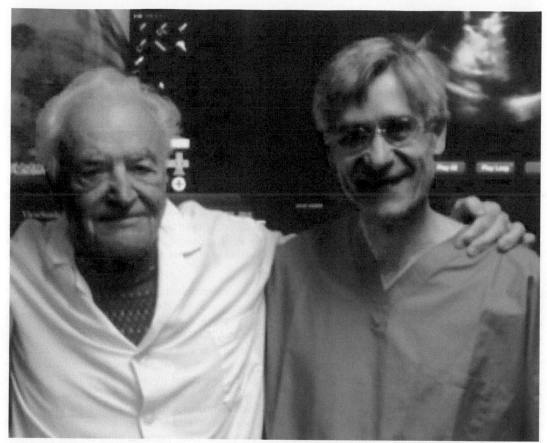

Fig. 6. Dog experiments. Kurt Amplatz (*left*) and the author in the catheterization laboratory during dog experiments with AMPLATZER left atrial appendage occlusions on April 3, 2008.

serial nonrandomized comparison.[28] Comparisons between the original ACP and the Amulet devices showed some advantages for Amulet in clinical results.[29–31] The Amulet showed good clinical results in a registry encompassing 1001 patients[32] with a 95% relative reduction of stroke (5.6% to 2.3%), when indirectly compared with anticoagulated patients with comparable risks scores, and a 61% reduction of bleeding (5.3% to 2.1%). The periprocedural complications amounted to 5.0%, most notably 1.3% cardiac tamponades, 0.9% strokes, and 0.8% procedure-related problems. Almost half of the interventions were done without echocardiographic guidance and particularly these

Table 1
Devices used in Europe for left atrial appendage occlusion

Device	Manufacturer	First Clinical Use
PLAATO[a]	EV3	2001
AMPLATZER (nondedicated)	AGA	June 15, 2002
WATCHMAN	Atritech/Boston Scientific	August 12, 2002
LAA TRANSCATHETER PATCH	Custom Medical Devices	2008
AMPLATZER Cardiac Plug/AMPLATZER Amulet	St. Jude/Abbott	2008
WAVECREST	Biosense Webster	2011
OCCLUTECH	Occlutech	2015
ULTRASEPT	Cardia	2015
LAmbre	Lifetech	2016

[a] No longer available.

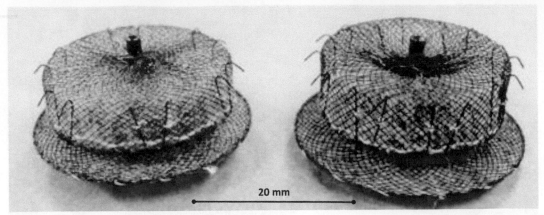

20 mm

Fig. 7. Dedicated AMPLATZER devices. AMPLATZER Cardiac Plug (*left*) and Amulet (*right*), the first- and second-generation dedicated AMPLATZER devices for left atrial appendage occlusion, consisting of nitinol wire braiding filled with absorbable polyester patches. (*Courtesy of* St. Jude Medical, Inc, Virginia Beach, VA; with permission.)

patients had many associated procedures. For instance, percutaneous coronary intervention, occlusion of an ASD or a patent foramen ovale, mitral valvuloplasty, septal reduction by alcohol, or left atrial ablation were performed simultaneously. The results were in keeping with the long-term results of the PROTECT AF randomized trial using the WATCHMAN device,[33] which had shown a mortality benefit compared with conservative treatment with warfarin in 707 patients eligible to both therapy modalities. In a propensity matched comparison, a survival benefit was also found in patients treated with AMPLATZER LAA occlusions in comparison with similar patients treated with oral anticoagulation (151 patients per group).[34] In the control group, 51% of patients were treated with antiplatelets, 17% with vitamin K antagonists, and 4% with non–vitamin K dependent oral anticoagulants. Per 1000 patient-years the mortality was reduced by 89% (hazard ratio, 0.16; confidence interval, 0.07–0.37). When using only patients on oral anticoagulation as comparator, mortality reduction was still 70% but it was no longer significant.

Modern global registries with about 1000 patients each showed a technical success rate of 99% with both the Amulet[35] and the WATCHMAN devices.[36] The major complication rates were 3.1% and 2.7%, respectively.

SUMMARY

Randomized data with WATCHMAN devices compellingly unveil LAA occlusion as superior to oral anticoagulation with warfarin even in terms of mortality, as early as a few years after the intervention. Indirect comparisons show that LAA occlusion with AMPLATZER devices is also competitive to non–vitamin K dependent oral anticoagulants.[37] A significant dependence of results on the device used is unlikely, at least among the two market leaders, AMPLATZER and WATCHMAN.[32,35,36] A respective randomized trial is currently recruiting patients. Every patient with atrial fibrillation should be thoroughly informed about the option of catheter-based LAA occlusion and these outcome data. Those who consent should undergo the procedure unless their life expectancy is shorter than a few years. Even patients who do not yet absolutely need oral anticoagulation (young healthy people with paroxysmal atrial fibrillation) may be candidates for LAA occlusion because their risk pattern will inevitably deteriorate and the risk of LAA occlusion is confined to the intervention and the early postintervention period. Guidelines[38] have to be adapted and the reimbursement has to be facilitated to make this progress in prevention of stroke and bleeding in patients with atrial fibrillation accessible for all, in the sense of a mechanical vaccination.

REFERENCES

1. Wolf PA, Abbott RD, Kannel WB. Atrial fibrillation as an independent risk factor for stroke: the Framingham Study. Stroke 1991;22:983–8.
2. Blackshear JL, Odell JA. Appendage obliteration to reduce stroke in cardiac surgical patients with atrial fibrillation. Ann Thorac Surg 1996;61:755–9.
3. Lin H, Wolf P, Kelly-Hayes M, et al. Stroke severity in atrial fibrillation. The Framingham Study. Stroke 1996;27:1760–4.
4. Marini C, De Santis F, Sacco S, et al. Contribution of atrial fibrillation to incidence and outcome of ischemic stroke: results from a population-based study. Stroke 2005;36:1115–9.

5. Al-Khatib SM, Thomas L, Wallentin L, et al. Outcomes of apixaban vs. warfarin by type and duration of atrial fibrillation: results from the ARISTOTLE trial. Eur Heart J 2013;34:2464–71.

6. Vanassche T, Lauw M, Eikelboom J, et al. Risk of ischaemic stroke according to pattern of atrial fibrillation: analysis of 6563 aspirin-treated patients in ACTIVE-A and AVERROES. Eur Heart J 2015;36: 281–287a.

7. Steinberg BA, Hellkamp AS, Lokhnygina Y, et al. Higher risk of death and stroke in patients with persistent vs. paroxysmal atrial fibrillation: results from the ROCKET-AF Trial. Eur Heart J 2015;36: 288–96.

8. Lip GY, Skjoth F, Rasmussen LH, et al. Oral anticoagulation, aspirin, or no therapy in patients with nonvalvular AF with 0 or 1 stroke risk factor based on the CHA2DS2-VASc score. J Am Coll Cardiol 2015;65:1385–94.

9. Sievert H, Lesh M, Trepels T, et al. Percutaneous left atrial appendage transcatheter occlusion to prevent stroke in high-risk patients with atrial fibrillation: early clinical experience. Circulation 2002; 105:1887–9.

10. Cox JL, Schuessler RB, D'Agostino HJJ, et al. The surgical treatment of atrial fibrillation. III. Development of a definitive surgical procedure. J Thorac Cardiovasc Surg 1991;101:569–83.

11. Cox JL, Ad N, Palazzo T. Impact of the maze procedure on the stroke rate in patients with atrial fibrillation. J Thorac Cardiovasc Surg 1999;118:833–40.

12. Schneider B, Stollberger C, Sievers HH. Surgical closure of the left atrial appendage: a beneficial procedure? Cardiology 2005;104:127–32.

13. Gillinov AM, Petterson G, Cosgrove DM. Stapled excision of the left atrial appendage. J Thorac Cardiovasc Surg 2005;129:679–80.

14. Jayakar D, Gozo F, Gomez E, et al. Use of tissue welding technology to obliterate left atrial appendage: novel use of Ligasure. Interact Cardiovasc Thorac Surg 2005;4:372–3.

15. Healey J, Crystal E, Lamy A, et al. Left Atrial Appendage Occlusion Study (LAAOS): results of a randomized controlled pilot study of left atrial appendage occlusion during coronary bypass surgery in patients at risk for stroke. Am Heart J 2005;150:288–93.

16. Kanderian AS, Gillinov AM, Pettersson GB, et al. Success of surgical left atrial appendage closure: assessment by transesophageal echocardiography. J Am Coll Cardiol 2008;52:924–9.

17. Salzberg SP, Plass A, Emmert MY, et al. Left atrial appendage clip occlusion: early clinical results. J Thorac Cardiovasc Surg 2010;139: 1269–74.

18. Benussi S, Mazzone P, Maccabelli G, et al. Thoracoscopic appendage exclusion with an atriclip device as a solo treatment for focal atrial tachycardia. Circulation 2011;123:1575–8.

19. Chatterjee S, Alexander JC, Pearson PJ, et al. Left atrial appendage occlusion: lessons learned from surgical and transcatheter experiences. Ann Thorac Surg 2011;92:2283–92.

20. Ailawadi G, Gerdisch MW, Harvey RL, et al. Exclusion of the left atrial appendage with a novel device: early results of a multicenter trial. J Thorac Cardiovasc Surg 2011;142:1002–9, 1009.e1.

21. Emmert MY, Puippe G, Baumuller S, et al. Safe, effective and durable epicardial left atrial appendage clip occlusion in patients with atrial fibrillation undergoing cardiac surgery: first long-term results from a prospective device trial. Eur J Cardiothorac Surg 2014;45:126–31.

22. Melduni RM, Schaff HV, Lee HC, et al. Impact of left atrial appendage closure during cardiac surgery on the occurrence of early postoperative atrial fibrillation, stroke, and mortality: a propensity score-matched analysis of 10 633 patients. Circulation 2017;135:366–78.

23. Praz F, Wahl A, Schmutz M, et al. Safety, feasibility, and long-term results of percutaneous closure of atrial septal defects using the Amplatzer septal occluder without periprocedural echocardiography. J Invasive Cardiol 2015;27:157–62.

24. Meier B, Palacios I, Windecker S, et al. Transcatheter left atrial appendage occlusion with Amplatzer devices to obviate anticoagulation in patients with atrial fibrillation. Catheter Cardiovasc Interv 2003; 60:417–22.

25. Meier B. Amplatzer devices for left atrial appendage occluders. In: Sievert H, Qureshi S, Wilson N, et al, editors. Percutaneous intervention for congenital heart disease. London: Informa Healthcare; 2007. p. 579–87.

26. Rodes-Cabau J, Champagne J, Bernier M. Transcatheter closure of the left atrial appendage: initial experience with the Amplatzer cardiac plug device. Catheter Cardiovasc Interv 2010;76:186–92.

27. Freixa X, Abualsaud A, Chan J, et al. Left atrial appendage occlusion: initial experience with the Amplatzer Amulet. Int J Cardiol 2014;174:492–6.

28. Schmid M, Gloekler S, Saguner A, et al. Transcatheter left atrial appendage closure in patients with atrial fibrillation: comparison between non-dedicated Amplatzer devices. Cardiovasc Med 2013;16:123–30.

29. Gloekler S, Shakir S, Doblies J, et al. Early results of first versus second generation Amplatzer occluders for left atrial appendage closure in patients with atrial fibrillation. Clin Res Cardiol 2015;104:656–65.

30. Abualsaud A, Freixa X, Tzikas A, et al. Side-by-side comparison of LAA occlusion performance with the Amplatzer Cardiac Plug and Amplatzer Amulet. J Invasive Cardiol 2016;28:34–8.

31. Al-Kassou B, Omran H. Comparison of the feasibility and safety of first- versus second-generation AMPLATZERC occluders for left atrial appendage closure. Biomed Res Int 2017;2017: 1519362.
32. Tzikas A, Shakir S, Gafoor S, et al. Left atrial appendage occlusion for stroke prevention in atrial fibrillation: multicentre experience with the AMPLATZER Cardiac Plug. EuroIntervention 2016; 11:1170–9.
33. Reddy VY, Sievert H, Halperin J, et al. Percutaneous left atrial appendage closure vs warfarin for atrial fibrillation: a randomized clinical trial. JAMA 2014; 312:1988–98.
34. Nielsen-Kudsk JE, Johnsen SP, Wester P, et al. Left atrial appendage occlusion versus standard medical care in patients with atrial fibrillation and intracerebral haemorrhage: a propensity score-matched follow-up study. EuroIntervention 2017; 13:371–8.
35. Landmesser U, Schmidt B, Nielsen-Kudsk JE, et al. Left atrial appendage occlusion with the AMPLATZER Amulet device: peri-procedural and early clinical/transoesophageal echocardiographic data ROM a global prospective registry. EuroIntervention 2017;13:867–76.
36. Boersma LV, Schmidt B, Betts TR, et al, EWOLUTION Investigators. Implant success and safety of left atrial appendage closure with the WATCHMAN device: peri-procedural outcomes from the EWOLUTION registry. Eur Heart J 2016;37:2465–74.
37. Nietlispach F, Gloekler S, Krause R, et al. Amplatzer left atrial appendage occlusion: single center 10-year experience. Catheter Cardiovasc Interv 2013;82:283–9.
38. Meier B, Blaauw Y, Khattab AA, et al. EHRA/EAPCI expert consensus statement on catheter-based left atrial appendage occlusion. Europace 2014;16: 1397–416.

Left Atrial Appendage Occlusion: Data Update

Matthew J. Price, MD

KEYWORDS

- Left atrial appendage • Atrial fibrillation • Thromboembolism • WATCHMAN
- Oral anticoagulation • Amulet

KEY POINTS

- Meta-analysis of the long-term follow-up of the PROTECT-AF and PREVAIL trials demonstrate that, compared with long-term warfarin, WATCHMAN LAA closure significantly reduces the composite endpoint of cardiovascular death, stroke, or systemic embolism, and reduces hemorrhagic stroke and all cause mortality.
- Pooled analyses of the WATCHMAN trials shows a significant reduction in major bleeding compared with warfarin once the post-implant pharmacologic regimen is completed.
- Observational data confirms improved procedural safety for WATCHMAN LAA closure since the early research experience.
- The AMULET randomized trial will evaluate whether the efficacy of Amulet LAA occluder is non-inferior to the WATCHMAN device.
- Further studies are required to define the optimal post-implant medical regimen to minimize device thrombus and bleeding, to clarify the relative efficacy of LAA closure compared with non-vitamin K oral anticoagulation, and to robustly demonstrate, in a randomized fashion, the safety and efficacy of LAA closure in patients who are ineligible for oral anticoagulation.

INTRODUCTION

Resection of the left atrial appendage (LAA) to prevent recurrent arterial emboli in patients with atrial fibrillation (AF) was first suggested more than 60 years ago,[1] and concomitant exclusion or removal of the LAA during cardiac surgery in high-risk patients with AF is now commonplace. More than a decade and a half has passed since small observational experiences reported the feasibility of transcatheter LAA occlusion.[2] However, longer-term follow-up from randomized studies of the safety and efficacy of LAA occlusion have only recently been completed; data from large, observational cohorts are now being reported. These recent data provide further insights into procedural safety with current techniques and the ability of LAA closure to reduce the risk of thromboembolic stroke compared with warfarin anticoagulation. This review summarizes the latest data regarding transcatheter LAA occlusion, focusing on larger prospective studies and further analyses of seminal clinical trials.

DATA FOR THE WATCHMAN LEFT ATRIAL APPENDAGE OCCLUDER

The WATCHMAN device (Boston Scientific, Natick, Massachusetts) is a parachute-shaped self-expanding device consisting of a nitinol frame and a polyethylene terephthalate fabric membrane cap that faces the body of the left atrium. Small tines that project back toward the left atrium line the circumference of the distal portion of the device that, in combination with radial force, anchor the device within the LAA.[3] The device was approved by the US Food and Drug Administration (FDA) because of the results from 2 randomized clinical trials, the PROTECT-AF

Division of Cardiovascular Diseases, Scripps Clinic, 9898 Genesee Avenue, AMP-200, La Jolla, CA 92037, USA
E-mail address: price.matthew@scrippshealth.org

Intervent Cardiol Clin 7 (2018) 159–168
https://doi.org/10.1016/j.iccl.2017.12.002

(WATCHMAN Left Atrial Appendage System for Embolic Protection in Patients with Atrial Fibrillation) study[4] and the smaller PREVAIL (Prospective Randomized Evaluation of the WATCHMAN Left Atrial Appendage Closure Device In Patients with Atrial Fibrillation vs Long-term Warfarin Therapy)[5] study, as well as the respective trials' continuing access registries. All of these studies enrolled patients with AF at higher risk of thromboembolism who were eligible for long-term oral anticoagulant therapy. More recent data regarding the WATCHMAN device include the final, 4-year follow-up from PROTECT-AF,[6] pooled patient-level meta-analyses of the two randomized trials,[7,8] and large prospective observational cohorts of WATCHMAN LAA closure in clinical practice.[9,10] These studies provide additional information regarding device safety and long-term bleeding, longer-term efficacy, the use of alternative post-implant pharmacologic regimens, procedural event rates in the commercial setting, and the feasibility of WATCHMAN LAA occlusion in patients who are ineligible for short- or long-term oral anticoagulant therapy.

Late Outcomes of the PROTECT-AF Trial

The PROTECT-AF trial randomly assigned 707 patients with AF with a CHADS$_2$ (congestive heart failure, hypertension, age ≥75 years, diabetes mellitus, and stroke/transient ischemic attack) score of 1 or greater who were eligible for long-term oral anticoagulant to either WATCHMAN LAA closure or warfarin in a 2:1 ratio.[4] The primary end point was a composite of cardiovascular or unexplained death, stroke, or systemic embolism. Patients who received the WATCHMAN device were continued on warfarin therapy for 6 weeks after the procedure, at which time they were transitioned to dual antiplatelet therapy with aspirin and clopidogrel for 5 months followed by indefinite aspirin maintenance therapy if LAA sealing was confirmed by transesophageal echocardiography (TEE) (Fig. 1). This

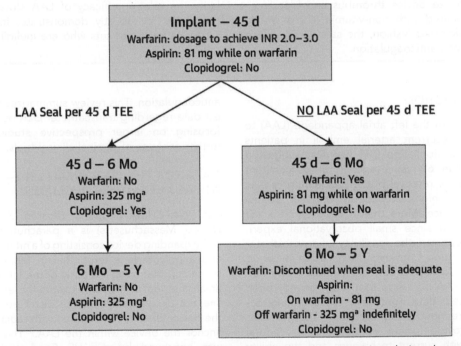

Fig. 1. Anticoagulant and antiplatelet management strategy in patients receiving device therapy in the PROTECT-AF and PREVAIL randomized clinical trials of the WATCHMAN LAA occluder. After device implantation, patients were treated with a combination of warfarin and aspirin for approximately 6 weeks, at which time TEE was performed. If the LAA was sealed (defined as a residual leak <5 mm in width without evidence of thrombus), warfarin was discontinued and the patients were treated with aspirin and clopidogrel until 6 months after the procedure, at which time the clopidogrel was discontinued and patients were continued on aspirin monotherapy. In the PROTECT-AF trial, patients could also receive clopidogrel at study entry if clinically indicated. [a]Recommended dosage. INR, international normalized ratio. (Adapted from Holmes DR, Jr, Kar S, Price MJ et al. Prospective randomized evaluation of the WATCHMAN left atrial appendage closure device in patients with atrial fibrillation vs long-term warfarin therapy: the PREVAIL trial. J Am Coll Cardiol 2014;64:3; with permission.)

protocol for postimplant therapy was followed across the WATCHMAN studies performed for FDA approval.

At a mean follow-up of 3.8 ± 1.7 years (2625 patient-years), LAA closure was both non-inferior and superior to warfarin for the primary efficacy end point (rate ratio, 0.60 [95% credible interval (CrI), 0.41–1.05], posterior probability of noninferiority greater than 99.9%, posterior probability for superiority = 96%). Both cardiovascular and all-cause mortality were reduced with LAA closure (hazard ratio [HR] 0.40 [95% confidence interval (CI), 0.21–0.75], P = .005 and HR 0.66 [95% CI, 0.45–0.98], P = .04, respectively). The rate of safety events, driven by procedural complications, was initially higher in the device group, although by the end of the follow-up the overall rates of safety events in both arms were similar, primarily due to the accrual of bleeding events in the warfarin group.

Late Follow Up of the PREVAIL Trial

The aim of the smaller PREVAIL trial was to confirm procedural safety, particularly among newer operators, and to further explore clinical efficacy of LAA closure compared with warfarin. The trial enrolled 407 AF patients with CHADS2 ≥2 who were randomly assigned to either WATCHMAN LAA closure or warfarin in a 2:1 ratio, and used a similar primary endpoint as PROTECT-AF.). The final results of PREVAIL, at a total follow-up of 1,626 patient-years, was recently reported. LAA closure with the WATCHMAN device met the performance goal for procedural and device safety pre-specified by the sponsor and the FDA, with safety events occurring in 2.2% of patients. The rate of ischemic stroke or systemic embolism > 7 days post-randomization was non-inferior with the WATCHMAN device compared with warfarin therapy, supporting the mechanistic hypothesis of LAA closure. The rate of the cardiovascular/unexplained death, stroke, or systemic embolism was was 0.065 in the device group versus 0.051 in the warfarin group, yielding a mean 18-month rate ratio of 1.32 (95% credible interval: 0.77 to 2.12). Given the wide 95% credible intervals, the trial was inconclusive regarding whether the efficacy of device therapy was non-inferior to long-term warfarin. Although none of the components of the primary efficacy endpoint were significantly different between treatment arms, the primary driver of failure to reach non-inferiority was a lower-than expected ischemic stroke rate in the warfarin group.[11]

PROTECT-AF and PREVAIL Meta-analysis

A meta-analysis of pooled, patient-level data from the PROTECT-AF and the smaller PREVAIL trial further assessed the outcomes of LAA closure with the WATCHMAN compared with warfarin in oral anticoagulation-eligible patients with AF.[11] In the meta-analysis, which combined PROTECT-AF at a mean follow-up of 47.6 ± 21.3 months and PREVAIL at a mean follow-up of 47.9 ± 19.4 months, the rate of the primary efficacy end point was similar with device closure and continued warfarin therapy (HR 0.82; 95% CI, 0.58–1.17; P = .27). All-cause stroke and systemic embolism were also similar with LAA closure and warfarin (HR 0.96, 95% CI, 0.60–1.54, P = .87); there was a trend for more ischemic strokes in the device group, significantly fewer hemorrhagic strokes in the warfarin group, and significantly fewer cardiovascular deaths in the device group (HR 0.59, 95% CI, 0.37–0.94; P = .27). The numerically higher rates of ischemic stroke in the device arm may have in part been due to a lower-than-expected ischemic stroke rate in the control arm of PREVAIL (despite a mean CHA_2DS_2-VASc [Congestive Heart failure, hypertension, Age ≥75 (doubled), Diabetes, Stroke (doubled), Vascular disease, Age 65–74, and Sex (female)] score of 4.0 ± 1.2) and several strokes due to air emboli during device deployment in the early part of PROTECT-AF. This numerical difference in ischemic stroke should be taken into context, as the rate of disabling stroke was significantly lower with WATCHMAN LAA closure compared with warfarin therapy (HR 0.45, 95% CI, 0.21–0.94; P = .034). Another pooled analysis of PROTECT-AF and PREVAIL demonstrated a significant reduction in major bleeding with LAA closure once the 6-month period of postprocedure pharmacotherapy was completed (1.0 events vs 3.5 events per 100 patient-years; Relative Risk 0.28; 95% CI, 0.16–0.49; P<.001), driven by reductions in gastrointestinal bleeding and intracranial hemorrhage (**Table 1, Fig. 2**).

ASAP Trial Long-Term Follow-up

The randomized clinical trials of WATCHMAN closure included patients who were eligible for oral anticoagulation, and the current FDA indication states that the WATCHMAN is only indicated in patients with AF who can tolerate short-term warfarin and have an appropriate rationale to seek a nonpharmacologic alternative. However, many patients with AF are simply not candidates for oral anticoagulation. ASAP

Table 1
Types and frequencies of postprocedural major bleeding events in the PROTECT-AF and PREVAIL trials

Bleeding Event	LAA Closure N = 732	Warfarin N = 382	P Value
Gastrointestinal bleeding, n (%)	10 (1.4%)	21 (5.5%)	<.001
Epistaxis, n (%)	1 (0.1%)	1 (0.3%)	1.0
Hematuria, n (%)	0 (0)	2 (0.5%)	.12
Hemorrhagic stroke, n (%)	2 (0.3%)	7 (1.8%)	.01
Cranial bleed, n (%)	3 (0.4%)	1 (0.3%)	1.0
Anemia requiring transfusion, n (%)	2 (0.3%)	1 (0.3%)	1.0
Major bleed requiring transfusion, n (%)	1 (0.1%)	1 (0.3%)	1.0
Other bleeding, n (%)	0 (0)	1 (0.3%)	.35

Bleeding events from the pooled PROTECT-AF and PREVAIL trials that occurred after the period of postimplant pharmacotherapy (oral anticoagulation and dual antiplatelet therapy) in the device group (>6 months after randomization).
Note that patients were randomly assigned to LAA closure or warfarin therapy in a 2:1 fashion.
Adapted from Price MJ, Reddy VY, Valderrabano M, et al. Bleeding outcomes after left atrial appendage closure compared with long-term warfarin: a pooled, patient-level analysis of the WATCHMAN randomized trial experience. JACC Cardiovasc Interv 2015;8:1925–32.

(ASA Plavix Feasibility Study with WATCHMAN Left Atrial Appendage Closure Technology) was a prospective, multicenter observational study that evaluated the safety and efficacy of WATCHMAN LAA closure in 150 patients with AF who were ineligible for warfarin therapy.[12,13] This patient population was not studied in the PROTECT-AF or PREVAIL randomized clinical trials. In ASAP, patients received dual antiplatelet therapy after implant with aspirin and clopidogrel for 6 months, then aspirin monotherapy thereafter. At a median follow-up of 55.4 months, the annual rate of ischemic stroke or systemic embolism was 1.8% (95% CI, 0.9% to 3.3%), which was approximately 75% lower than the expected rate in a hypothetical patient population with a similar $CHADS_2$ score treated with aspirin alone (**Fig. 3**). The role of WATCHMAN LAA closure in oral anticoagulation–contraindicated patients will be more robustly studied in the ASAP-TOO trial (Assessment of the WATCHMAN Device in Patients Unsuitable for Oral Anticoagulation) trial (clinicaltrials.gov identifier, NCT02928497). This prospective multicenter clinical trial will randomly assign approximately 900 patients

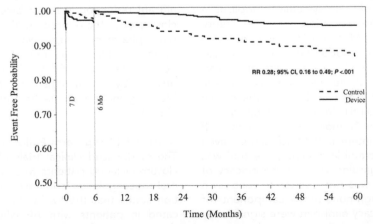

Fig. 2. Freedom from first major bleed from 6 months after randomization to the end of follow-up in a pooled, patient-level analysis of the PROTECT-AF and PREVAIL trials. (*Adapted from* Price MJ, Reddy VY, Valderrabano M, et al. Bleeding outcomes after left atrial appendage closure compared with long-term warfarin: a pooled, patient-level analysis of the WATCHMAN randomized trial experience. JACC Cardiovasc Interv 2015;8:1930; with permission.)

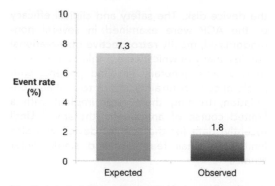

Fig. 3. Late incidence of ischemic stroke or systemic embolism in the ASAP study of WATCHMAN LAA occlusion compared with that expected with aspirin monotherapy in patients with AF who were unsuitable for oral anticoagulation. The observed rate of ischemic stroke or systemic embolism after LAA occlusion was substantially lower than the expected rate of a hypothetical population with similar thromboembolic risk treated with aspirin alone. (*Adapted from* Sharma D, Reddy VY, Sandri M et al. Left atrial appendage closure in patients with contraindications to oral anticoagulation. J Am Coll Cardiol 2016;67:2191; with permission.)

with AF who are deemed unsuitable to oral anticoagulation to either medical therapy (single or no antiplatelet therapy per operator discretion) or WATCHMAN LAA closure followed by a modified postimplant drug regimen of dual antiplatelet therapy.

Early WATCHMAN Commercial Experience
The observed rates of procedural complications significantly decreased over the course of the WATCHMAN clinical trial experience. In the initial PROTECT-AF trial, procedure-related adverse events at 7 days after the procedure occurred in 8.7% of patients, including pericardial tamponade requiring intervention in 4.0%.[4,7] In the subsequent PREVAIL trial, the WATCHMAN device met its prespecified criterion for procedural safety; the procedural complication rate was 4.5%, with 1.9% of patients having a pericardial effusion requiring intervention, substantially lower than that observed in PROTECT-AF.[5] Whether this improved procedural safety would be observed in the real world after commercial approval is an open question. To answer this, Reddy and colleagues[9] reported the procedural outcomes of the first cohort of patients who underwent WATCHMAN LAA closure in the US commercial setting. A total of 3822 patients were treated by 382 operators at 169 centers, and operators who were not involved in the prior clinical study experience performed approximately half the cases. The rate of

periprocedural complications was less than 1.5%: procedure-related death (all due to pericardial tamponade) occurred in 0.08%, procedure-related stroke in 0.08%, pericardial tamponade requiring intervention in 1.0%, and device embolization in 0.25% (two-thirds of which required surgical retrieval). Although these results confirm the safety of the WATCHMAN LAA closure in the early commercial experience, the study design may have led to underreporting of events because periprocedural events were collected and reported by the manufacturer's clinical specialists and events that occurred outside the catheterization laboratory may not have been fully captured.[14] The National Cardiovascular Data Registry Left Atrial Appendage Occlusion Registry will play a key role in understanding the safety of transcatheter LAA closure for stroke prevention as it is currently applied in the United States.

EWOLUTION Registry
The evolving procedural safety and longer-term efficacy of WATCHMAN LAA closure in the real world was also explored in the EWOLUTION registry.[10] In this prospective, multicenter, observational study, 1027 patients with AF at high thromboembolic risk and either eligible or ineligible for oral anticoagulation were enrolled at 47 sites outside of the United States. The average CHA_2DS_2-VASc score of the study population was 4.5 ± 1.6, and the average HAS-BLED (hypertension, abnormal renal/liver function [1 point each], stroke, bleeding history or predisposition, labile INR, elderly [>65 years], drugs/alcohol concomitantly [1 point each]) score was 2.3 ± 1.2; 61.8% of the patients were considered ineligible for oral anticoagulation. Serious procedure and/or device-related adverse events within the first 7 days after the procedure occurred in 2.7% of cases, lower than that observed in the prior randomized trials (Fig. 4). Procedural safety was consistent across important subgroups. Patients outside the United States are treated with a broad spectrum of postprocedure pharmacology, unlike those enrolled in the protocols that led to device approval by the FDA. In the EWOLUTION registry, 60% of patients were treated after the procedure with dual antiplatelet therapy, 16% with vitamin-K antagonists, 11% with non–vitamin K antagonists, 7% with single antiplatelet therapy, and 6% without either anticoagulation or antithrombotic therapy.[15] There were no differences in 3-month bleeding rates across these postprocedure drug regimens, although the numerically lowest rate occurred in the patients treated with non–vitamin K antagonists, who also happened to have the

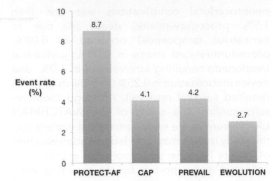

Fig. 4. Rates of serious procedure- and device-related events in the PROTECT-AF, Continued Access to PROTECT-AF (CAP), PREVAIL, and EWOLUTION. The available data suggest the procedural safety of transcatheter LAA occlusion has improved over time. (*Adapted from* Boersma LV, Schmidt B, Betts TR et al. Implant success and safety of left atrial appendage closure with the WATCHMAN device: peri-procedural outcomes from the EWOLUTION registry. Eur Heart J 2016;37(31):2465–74; with permission.)

lowest HAS-BLED scores. There were also no significant differences in the rates of device thrombosis at the time of follow-up TEE, although the highest rate was observed in the group of patients treated with dual antiplatelet therapy. Of note, the robustness of these comparisons is limited, as they are underpowered; furthermore, the choice of postimplant pharmacology was not randomized and the baseline characteristics of the groups getting the various regimens differed substantially; therefore, the comparisons are subject to substantial confounding.

AMULET LEFT ATRIAL APPENDAGE OCCLUDER

The Amplatzer Amulet (St Jude Medical, Minneapolis, Minnesota) is a second-generation iteration of the Amplatzer Cardiac Plug (ACP). The device consists of a self-expanding nitinol mesh that forms a distal lobe and proximal disk, each with a sewn polyester patch, connected by a short central waist. The distal lobe has stabilizing wires around its circumference that together with the self-expanding force of the lobe anchors the device within the LAA, whereas the proximal disk covers the mouth of the LAA from within the left atrium akin to a baby pacifier.[16] The mechanism of LAA occlusion, thus, differs from that of the WATCHMAN as the Amulet provides 2 potential layers of LAA closure, one at the level of the device lobe and a second at the level of the device disk. The safety and clinical efficacy of the ACP were examined in several non-randomized, mostly retrospective observational studies, many of which were single-center experiences, and generally enrolled patients with intolerance or contraindications to oral anticoagulation, treating them after implant with a limited course of antiplatelet therapy.[17] Until recently, data for the Amulet device was also limited to small feasibility and single-center studies.[18–20]

Amulet Global Observational Registry
A large prospective, observational experience with an independent clinical events committee was recently reported.[21] In this prospective registry, 1088 patients were enrolled at 61 sites in Europe, Australia, Israel, Chile, and Hong Kong. The study population was at a high thromboembolic and bleeding risk: the mean $CHA_2DS_2\text{-VASc}$ score was 4.2 ± 1.6; the mean HAS-BLED score was 3.3 ± 1.1; the HAS-BLED score was 3 or more in 78%. Unlike the patients evaluated in the WATCHMAN research experience, who were eligible for long-term oral anticoagulation, 83% of the patients enrolled in this global registry had contraindications to oral anticoagulation. Amulet implantation was technically successful (successful implantation of the device in the correct position) in 99% of cases, and procedural success (technical success without major procedural complication) was achieved in 95.8% of cases. Major procedural complications occurred in 3.2% of patients (95% CI, 2.2%–4.4%), including pericardial effusion or tamponade in 1.2%, vascular complication in 0.9%, periprocedural stroke in 0.2%, and death in 0.2%. Periprocedural device embolization occurred in only 1 patient (0.1%). At discharge, most patients (54.0%) were treated with dual antiplatelet therapy, whereas a minority was treated with oral anticoagulation (18.9%), single antiplatelet therapy (23.0%), or no antiplatelet or oral anticoagulation (2.0%).

Follow-up TEE imaging was available in 673 patients (62%) at a mean of 2.4 ±0.8 months after implant. A peri-device leak less than 3 mm was rarely observed (1.8%), and device thrombus was identified in 1.5%. There was one late device embolization (0.1%), which was retrieved successfully using a percutaneous approach. The composite end point of cardiovascular death, ischemic stroke, or systemic embolism beyond 7 days after the procedure and within 3 months of implant occurred in 15 patients (1.4%, 95%

CI, 0.8%–2.3%), driven by cardiovascular death (13 patients).

In sum, this prospective global experience supports the hypothesis that transcatheter LAA closure is associated with a relatively low rate of procedural events and device-related thrombosis, with complication rates generally similar or less than those observed in the randomized clinical trials for the WATCHMAN device. These data are more robust than the evidence base for the ACP device, given its prospective, multicenter design with an independent core laboratory and clinical events committee. However, any conclusions about device thrombosis need to be tempered by the many patients in whom surveillance TEE was not available, raising the possibility of selection bias. Further clinical follow-up is required to assess efficacy with respect to stroke reduction, which will need to be interpreted through imputed placebo comparisons, that is, by comparing with the expected thromboembolic rates in a similar population not treated with the Amulet. However, such comparisons have methodological limitations and are not as robust as a randomized clinical trial.

Several randomized trials of the Amulet device are either planned or ongoing. The STROKECLOSE (Prevention of Stroke by Left Atrial Appendage Closure in Atrial Fibrillation Patients After Intracerebral Hemorrhage) trial (clinicaltrials.gov identifier, NCT02830152) will randomly assign 750 patients with AF with prior intracranial hemorrhage in a 2:1 fashion to Amulet LAA occlusion or medical therapy; the primary end point is the composite of any stroke, major bleeding, and death at 2 years. The AMULET LAA Occluder trial (clinicaltrials.gov identifier, NCT02879448) is a prospective, randomized, noninferiority trial of the Amulet versus the WATCHMAN LAA occluder in approximately 1600 patients with AF at high thromboembolic risk who are deemed suitable for short-term warfarin but not good candidates for long-term oral anticoagulation. Three primary outcomes will be measured: device closure at 45 days; safety (the composite of procedure-related complications, all-cause death, or major bleeding) at 1 year; and efficacy (stroke or systemic embolism) at 18 months.

DEVICE THROMBUS

The development of thrombus on the surface of the LAA occluder is of significant clinical concern. Device thrombus might place patients at very high risk of thromboembolic events and require treatment with oral anticoagulation, both sequelae that the LAA closure procedure was designed to avoid in the first place. The identification of risk factors that predispose to device thrombus could also help inform the optimal postimplant medication regimen and the appropriate intensity for surveillance with TEE or computed tomography. Lempereur and colleagues[22] performed a systematic review of reported device thrombus in 30 studies involving the ACP, the Amulet, and the WATCHMAN occluders. The overall incidence of device thrombus was 3.9% at a median follow-up of 1.5 months. Device thrombus was treated successfully (ie, complete thrombus resolution) in almost all cases (95%) with a treatment course of either low molecular heparin (100% success) or oral coagulation (90% success) over a median of 45 days (interquartile range, 14–135 days). Saw and colleagues[23] reported the incidence and sequelae of device thrombus in the retrospective, ACP multicenter experience, which enrolled 1047 patients undergoing LAA closure with the ACP at 22 centers outside of the United States.[17] Surveillance TEEs were available for independent review from 339 of the 1019 patients with successful ACP implantation (33.3%) at a median follow-up of 134 days (range, 179–622 days). The type of postimplant therapy was available in 255 patients, most of which was dual antiplatelet therapy. Device thrombus was noted in 3.2% of cases, none of which was associated with a thromboembolic event. Only smoking and female sex were independently associated with the presence of device thrombus.

The Lariat device (SentreHeart, Redwood City, California) enables the percutaneous ligation of the LAA through the delivery of a surgical suture via a combined transseptal and subxiphoid approach.[3] Frequent residual and late leaks after this procedure have been reported.[24] In a retrospective multicenter study of 98 patients undergoing Lariat LAA ligation, leaks were present in 20% of cases.[25] There were 3 patients with late stroke (>6 months after the procedure), all of whom had small leaks into the LAA (<5 mm in diameter). This study emphasizes the importance of surveillance TEE post-Lariat LAA ligation, and that the optimal post-Lariat antiplatelet or anticoagulation regimen remains to be defined. Transcatheter occlusion of post-Lariat LAA leaks with occluder devices is feasible, but the long-term efficacy of this approach in terms of stroke prevention is unknown.[26]

EVIDENCE GAPS

Significant evidence gaps remain despite the increased body of data examining the safety and efficacy of transcatheter LAA closure. The results of PROTECT-AF and PREVAIL suggest that occlusion of the LAA might be associated with a slightly higher risk of ischemic stroke compared with warfarin. There exist several benign explanations for this observation. For example, the rate of periprocedural stroke in the device arm of PROTECT-AF was much higher than observed in more recent experiences.[4,9,10] The event rate in the control (warfarin) arm of PREVAIL was remarkably lower than expected based on CHADS$_2$ and CHA$_2$DS$_2$-VASc scores. In patients at high thromboembolic risk (eg, elderly age, diabetes, renal dysfunction, heart failure, and/or peripheral vascular disease), long-term oral anticoagulation may reduce ischemic events independently of AF-related mechanisms. Unfortunately, because the upcoming pivotal trials of novel devices use noninferiority designs versus the WATCHMAN device, future randomized controlled trials sufficiently powered to compare the efficacy of transcatheter LAA occlusion with long-term oral anticoagulation are unlikely to be performed; therefore, efficacy will have to be gleaned from the absolute event rates in large, prospective experiences, possibly by comparing these rates with an imputed placebo. Similarly, the randomized clinical trials that have been performed did not compare LAA occlusion with non–vitamin K oral anticoagulants, which are easier to use and generally safer than warfarin. A network meta-analysis suggested that both non–vitamin K antagonists and WATCHMAN were superior to warfarin for preventing hemorrhagic strokes, non–vitamin K antagonists were superior to warfarin for reducing all-cause stroke and major bleeding, and there were no significant differences in outcomes between non–vitamin K antagonists and WATCHMAN, although there was a trend for more ischemic stroke and less hemorrhagic stroke with WATCHMAN.[27] The relative safety and efficacy of LAA closure compared with non–vitamin K antagonist therapy will be explored by the PRAGUE-17 study (Left Atrial Appendage Closure vs Novel Anticoagulation Agents in Atrial Fibrillation), which will randomize approximately 400 patients with AF to either non–vitamin K oral anticoagulant

therapy or transcatheter LAA occlusion with the Amulet or WATCHMAN device (clinicaltrials.gov identifier, NCT02426944). The primary end point will combine both safety and efficacy, measuring the composite of stroke, other systemic cardio-embolic events, clinically significant bleeding, cardiovascular death, or procedure/device-related complications at 1 year. This last study may be informative but will likely not provide definitive answers for efficacy given its small sample size and the composite nature of the primary end point.

SUMMARY

LAA occlusion is an important alternative to oral anticoagulation in patients with AF, particularly in those who are not good candidates for long-term therapy. Late follow-up from the PROTECT-AF and PREVAIL trials demonstrates substantial reductions in hemorrhagic stroke and cardiovascular death with WATCHMAN LAA closure compared with continued warfarin therapy. Pooled analyses of the WATCHMAN trials show a significant reduction in major bleeding compared with warfarin once the postimplant pharmacologic regimen is completed. A growing body of observational data confirms improved procedural safety for WATCHMAN LAA closure since the early research experience; the procedural safety of the Amulet device seems comparable, although this will be tested in the ongoing, randomized AMULET trial. Further studies are required to define the optimal postimplant medical regimen to minimize device thrombus and bleeding, to clarify the relative efficacy of LAA closure to prevent ischemic stroke compared with oral anticoagulation in eligible patients, and to robustly demonstrate, in a randomized fashion, the safety and efficacy of LAA closure in patients who are ineligible for oral anticoagulation.

REFERENCES

1. Madden JL. Resection of the left auricular appendix; a prophylaxis for recurrent arterial emboli. J Am Med Assoc 1949;140:769–72.
2. Sievert H, Lesh MD, Trepels T, et al. Percutaneous left atrial appendage transcatheter occlusion to prevent stroke in high-risk patients with atrial fibrillation: early clinical experience. Circulation 2002; 105:1887–9.
3. Price MJ, Valderrabano M. Left atrial appendage closure to prevent stroke in patients

with atrial fibrillation. Circulation 2014;130: 202–12.

4. Holmes DR, Reddy VY, Turi ZG, et al. Percutaneous closure of the left atrial appendage versus warfarin therapy for prevention of stroke in patients with atrial fibrillation: a randomised non-inferiority trial. Lancet 2009; 374:534–42.

5. Holmes DR Jr, Kar S, Price MJ, et al. Prospective randomized evaluation of the watchman left atrial appendage closure device in patients with atrial fibrillation versus long-term warfarin therapy: the PREVAIL trial. J Am Coll Cardiol 2014;64:1–12.

6. Reddy VY, Sievert H, Halperin J, et al. Percutaneous left atrial appendage closure vs warfarin for atrial fibrillation: a randomized clinical trial. JAMA 2014; 312:1988–98.

7. Holmes DR Jr, Doshi SK, Kar S, et al. Left atrial appendage closure as an alternative to warfarin for stroke prevention in atrial fibrillation: a patient-level meta-analysis. J Am Coll Cardiol 2015;65:2614–23.

8. Price MJ, Reddy VY, Valderrabano M, et al. Bleeding outcomes after left atrial appendage closure compared with long-term warfarin: a pooled, patient-level analysis of the WATCHMAN randomized trial experience. JACC Cardiovasc Interv 2015;8:1925–32.

9. Reddy VY, Gibson DN, Kar S, et al. Post-approval U.S. experience with left atrial appendage closure for stroke prevention in atrial fibrillation. J Am Coll Cardiol 2017;69:253–61.

10. Boersma LV, Schmidt B, Betts TR, et al. Implant success and safety of left atrial appendage closure with the WATCHMAN device: peri-procedural outcomes from the EWOLUTION registry. Eur Heart J 2016;37(31):2465–74.

11. Reddy VY, Doshi SK, Kar S, et al. 5-Year Outcomes After Left Atrial Appendage Closure: From the PREVAIL and PROTECT AF Trials. J Am Coll Cardiol 2017;70(24):2964–75.

12. Reddy VY, Mobius-Winkler S, Miller MA, et al. Left atrial appendage closure with the watchman device in patients with a contraindication for oral anticoagulation: the ASAP study (ASA Plavix feasibility study with watchman left atrial appendage closure technology). J Am Coll Cardiol 2013;61: 2551–6.

13. Sharma D, Reddy VY, Sandri M, et al. Left atrial appendage closure in patients with contraindications to oral anticoagulation. J Am Coll Cardiol 2016;67:2190–2.

14. Saw J, Price MJ. Assessing the safety of early U.S. commercial application of left atrial appendage closure. J Am Coll Cardiol 2017;69: 262–4.

15. Bergmann MW, Betts TR, Sievert H, et al. Early anticoagulation drug regimens after WATCHMAN left atrial appendage closure: safety and efficacy. EuroIntervention 2017;13(7): 877–84.

16. Tzikas A, Gafoor S, Meerkin D, et al. Left atrial appendage occlusion with the AMPLATZER amulet device: an expert consensus step-by-step approach. EuroIntervention 2016;11:1512–21.

17. Tzikas A, Shakir S, Gafoor S, et al. Left atrial appendage occlusion for stroke prevention in atrial fibrillation: multicentre experience with the AMPLATZER cardiac plug. EuroIntervention 2016; 11:1170–9.

18. Lam SC, Bertog S, Gafoor S, et al. Left atrial appendage closure using the amulet device: an initial experience with the second generation Amplatzer cardiac plug. Catheter Cardiovasc Interv 2015;85(2):297–303.

19. Freixa X, Abualsaud A, Chan J, et al. Left atrial appendage occlusion: initial experience with the Amplatzer amulet. Int J Cardiol 2014;174: 492–6.

20. Gloekler S, Shakir S, Doblies J, et al. Early results of first versus second generation Amplatzer occluders for left atrial appendage closure in patients with atrial fibrillation. Clin Res Cardiol 2015;104:656–65.

21. Landmesser U, Schmidt B, Nielsen-Kudsk JE, et al. Left atrial appendage occlusion with the AMPLATZER amulet device: periprocedural and early clinical/echocardiographic data from a global prospective observational study. EuroIntervention 2017;13(7): 867–76.

22. Lempereur M, Aminian A, Freixa X, et al. Device-associated thrombus formation after left atrial appendage occlusion: a systematic review of events reported with the watchman, the Amplatzer cardiac plug and the amulet. Catheter Cardiovasc Interv 2017;90(5): E111–21.

23. Saw J, Tzikas A, Shakir S, et al. Incidence and clinical impact of device-associated thrombus and peri-device leak following left atrial appendage closure with the Amplatzer cardiac plug. JACC Cardiovasc Interv 2017;10: 391–9.

24. Price MJ, Gibson DN, Yakubov SJ, et al. Early safety and efficacy of percutaneous left atrial appendage suture ligation: results from the U.S. transcatheter LAA ligation consortium. J Am Coll Cardiol 2014; 64:565–72.

25. Gianni C, Di Biase L, Trivedi C, et al. Clinical implications of leaks following left atrial appendage ligation with the LARIAT device. JACC Cardiovasc Interv 2016;9:1051–7.

26. Mosley WJ 2nd, Smith MR, Price MJ. Percutaneous management of late leak after lariat transcatheter ligation of the left atrial appendage in patients with atrial fibrillation at high risk for stroke. Catheter Cardiovasc Interv 2014;83:664–9.

27. Koifman E, Lipinski MJ, Escarcega RO, et al. Comparison of Watchman device with new oral anticoagulants in patients with atrial fibrillation: a network meta-analysis. Int J Cardiol 2016;205: 17–22.

Indication, Patient Selection, and Referral Pathways for Left Atrial Appendage Closure

Tawseef Dar, MD[a], Mohit K. Turagam, MD[b],
Bharath Yarlagadda, MD[a], Mohmad Tantary, MD[c],
Seth H. Sheldon, MD[d],
Dhanunjaya Lakkireddy, MD, FHRS[d],*

KEYWORDS

- Atrial fibrillation • Left atrial appendage • WATCHMAN • LARIAT • Amulet
- Thromboembolism • Anticoagulation

KEY POINTS

- Left atrial appendage closure (LAAC) is a viable alternative to oral anticoagulation therapy (OAC) for patients with nonvalvular atrial fibrillation who are considered poor candidates for long-term oral anticoagulation.
- Current consensus on LAAC indications, patient, and device selection.
- Patient selection for this procedure continues to evolve with growing expertise, technology, and ongoing clinical investigation on its use in various patient populations.
- We propose a model for appropriate referral system for patients undergoing LAAC for favorable clinical outcomes.

INTRODUCTION

Atrial fibrillation (AF) is the most common arrhythmia encountered by clinicians with evidence suggesting an increasing prevalence and incidence worldwide.[1-3] Thromboembolic stroke related to AF with associated morbidity and mortality remains a challenge for diverse reasons.[4] One of the main challenges is the risk of bleeding associated with pharmacotherapy. The incidence of AF, risk of stroke, and risk of bleeding increase with age, creating a difficult situation. The overall prevalence of AF is 1%. Out of all patients with AF, 70% are 65 and older and 45% are 75 years and older, respectively. The prevalence of AF ranged from 0.1% among adults less than 55 years of age to 9% in those 80 years of age and older.[5] In the setting of nonvalvular AF, 90% of thrombi are located within the left atrial appendage (LAA).[6] Left atrial fibrosis and inflammation in patients with AF is particularly intense in the LAA and may account for this finding. Oral anticoagulation therapy (vitamin K antagonists [VKA] or non-VKA oral anticoagulants [NOAC]) has long been used for prevention of thromboembolism in patients with AF and remains the first-line

Disclosures: The authors have nothing to disclose.
[a] Division of Cardiovascular Diseases, Cardiovascular Research Institute, University of Kansas Hospital and Medical Center, 3901 Rainbow Boulevard, Kansas City, KS 66160, USA; [b] Division of Cardiology, Helmsey Center for Electrophysiology, Icahn School of Medicine at Mount Sinai, 1190 5th Avenue, 1 South, New York, NY 10029, USA; [c] Department of Internal Medicine, Clinch Valley Medical Center, 6801 Governor G C Peery Highway, Richlands, VA 24641, USA; [d] Division of Cardiovascular Diseases, Cardiovascular Research Institute, University of Kansas Hospital and Medical Center, 3901 Rainbow Boulevard, Kansas City, KS 66160, USA
* Correspondent author.
E-mail address: dlakkireddy@kumc.edu

Intervent Cardiol Clin 7 (2018) 169–183
https://doi.org/10.1016/j.iccl.2017.12.003
2211-7458/18/© 2017 Elsevier Inc. All rights reserved.

therapy.[7,8] In some patients, challenges arise either starting or continuing oral anticoagulation (OAC) therapy. Patients are at increased risk of bleeding events secondary to OAC therapy, especially life-threatening intracranial hemorrhage (ICH) and gastrointestinal bleeding. In the past decade, NOACs have emerged as a safer and more effective alternative than VKA[9–12] but the risk of bleeding with anticoagulation remains because the risk factors for thromboembolism and bleeding are largely driven by an overlapping set of comorbidities.[13] Approximately 50% of patients with AF who have a guideline indication for OAC therapy end up not being on any form of OAC therapy for diverse reasons.[14] In recent years, there has been a focus on development and implementation of nonpharmacologic measures to prevent cardioembolic events and fulfill a clinical need for a significant proportion of patients. LAA occlusion, including endocardial and epicardial devices, has emerged as an attractive and promising alternative to OAC therapy.

METHODS OF LEFT ATRIAL APPENDAGE CLOSURE AND CLINICAL EVIDENCE SUPPORTING LEFT ATRIAL APPENDAGE CLOSURE

Currently there are two main approaches for LAAC: surgical and percutaneous.

Surgical Methods/Approach

Surgical methods/approach includes open surgical approaches and minimally invasive thoracoscopic technique. In 2015, a meta-analysis of two randomized trials and five observational studies of surgical LAAC in the setting of cardiac surgery (n = 3653 patients) was done and showed that LAAC is associated with a lower incidence of stroke at 30-day follow-up (0.95 vs 1.9%; odds ratio [OR], 0.46; P = .005) and last follow-up (1.4 vs 4.1%; OR, 0.48; P = .01).[15]

Based on available data, current European Society of Cardiology and American Heart Association/American College of Cardiology guidelines make a suggestion that surgical excision of the LAA may be considered in patients undergoing cardiac surgery or thoracoscopic AF surgery (grade IIb recommendation with level B and C evidence, respectively).[8,16]

Data from multiple studies, however, have raised concerns about efficacy of surgical LAAC techniques, especially suture exclusion. Kanderian and colleagues[17] reported an overall success rate of 40% for LAAC, with surgical excision achieving higher success rates (73%) than suture exclusion (23%), after a mean follow-up of

8.1 ± 12 months. Unsuccessful LAAC was defined as the presence of a patent LAA, excluded LAA with persistent flow, or a remnant LAA. An active LAA thrombus was present in 41% and 0% of unsuccessful LAA exclusion and excision, respectively. Cullen and colleagues,[18] in a retrospective 1-month follow-up data after surgical LAAC, showed a residual communication from LAA in 37% of cases with an active thrombus present in 28% of all patients and 47% of patients with incomplete LAAC. The safety of anticoagulation discontinuation in patients after surgical LAAC is uncertain, especially if a transesophageal echo (TEE) is not performed to confirm successful closure and the absence of an LAA thrombus.

Newer techniques, such as the epicardial AtriCure Atriclip system (Atricure, West Chester, OH) (Fig. 1), used during open or thoracoscopic surgery, have improved the success rates of LAA exclusion. A multicenter evaluation of the Atricure clip reported a more than 98% closure rate at 3-month follow-up TEE/computed tomography angiography.[19]

Percutaneous Methods/Approach
WATCHMAN device

The safety and efficacy of the WATCHMAN device (Boston Scientific Corp, Marlborough, MA) was evaluated in two randomized trials: the PROTECT AF study (Left Atrial Appendage System for Embolic Protection in Patients with Atrial Fibrillation) followed by the PREVAIL (Prospective Randomized Evaluation of the Watchman LAA Closure Device in Patients with Atrial Fibrillation vs Long-Term Warfarin Therapy) study (Fig. 2).[20–23]

The PREVAIL study and CAP registry reported an improvement in implant success rate (90.9% PROTECT AF to 94.3% CAP to 95.1% PREVAIL; P = .04) and a significant decline in iatrogenic complications (periprocedural) indicating improvement in operator experience and training with time. All 7-day procedural complication rates declined from 8.7% in PROTECT AF trial to 4.2% and 4.5% (P = .004), as reported from CAP and PREVAIL data, respectively. The rate of pericardial effusion requiring surgery dropped from 1.6% in PROTECT AF trial to 0.2% and 0.4% (P = .03) in CAP and PREVAIL data, respectively.[22]

Based on the results of PROTECT AF and PREVAIL, the WATCHMAN device was approved by the US Food and Drug Administration (FDA) in March 2015 for patients with nonvalvular AF for whom long-term anticoagulation is indicated, but who have a rational reason for not adhering to such therapy. These patients must be able to tolerate warfarin for at least

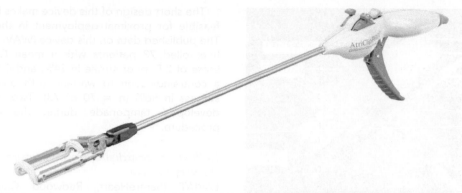

Fig. 1. Atriclip delivery system. (*Courtesy of* Atricure, West Chester, OH; with permission.)

6 weeks after the device is implanted and cannot have LAA clot present at the time of implantation.

A recent multicenter retrospective study suggests NOACs are a feasible alternative to warfarin for periprocedural and post-procedural anticoagulation, thereby avoiding the complexity of warfarin therapy.[24]

AMPLATZER cardiac plug/Amulet

The AMPLATZER cardiac plug (ACP) device has potentially advantageous features including a larger lobe size, more stabilizing wires to fit larger appendages, and a short waist between proximal left atrial disk and a distal LAA lobe to fit short appendages (Fig. 3).[25,26] This device has not yet received FDA approval. The ACP has a self-expanding nitinol frame forming a lobe and a disk with polyester fabric and peripheral fixation hooks. The proximal disk is meant to enhance the potential for complete closure, called the pacifier principle.[27]

The largest published data on ACP are from a multicenter study (n = 22 centers) that included 1047 patients with a mean $CHA_2DS_2\text{-}VASc$ score of 4, and 29% were on OAC. The procedural success rate was 97% with a periprocedural major adverse event rate of 5% (cardiac tamponade of 1.24% and major bleeding of 1.24% were the predominant ones). The annual stroke rate was 2.3% (31 of 1349 patient-years), which was 59% lower than expected based on patient risk scores.[28] ACP received CE Mark approval in Europe in 2008.

Amulet (Fig. 4), a second-generation device (with sizes up to 32 mm), is now available in Europe, and currently under postmarketing surveillance. It is also under investigation in a randomized trial in the United States. The main

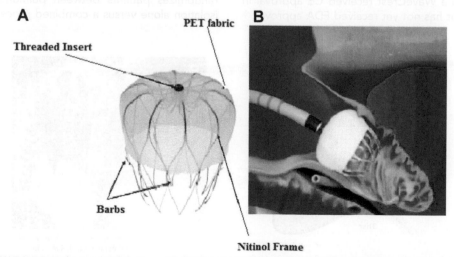

A
Threaded Insert
PET fabric
Barbs
Nitinol Frame

B

Fig. 2. WATCHMAN device. (*A*) Structure. (*B*) Inside left atrial appendage. PET, polyethyleneterphthalate. (Image provided *courtesy of* Boston Scientific. ©2018 Boston Scientific Corporation or its affiliates. All rights reserved.)

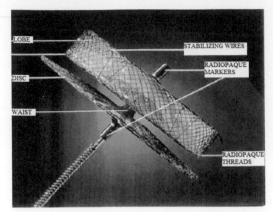

Fig. 3. AMPLATZER cardiac plug. (*Courtesy of* Abbott, Abbott Park, IL; with permission.)

advantage is a lower rate of any peridevice leaks compared with the ACP device (48% with ACP vs 8% with Amulet; $P = .01$) and less risk of dislodgment, as evident from small cohorts.[29,30] Amulet received CE Mark in 2013.

The AMPLATZER device is being evaluated in several randomized trials. The ELIGIBLE (efficacy of LAAC after gastrointestinal bleeding) will randomize 120 patients to AMPLATZER implantation and 3 months of aspirin and clopidogrel versus OAC in patients with prior gastrointestinal bleeding (ClinicalTrials.gov Identifier: NCT01628068).

WaveCrest device

The WaveCrest LAA occluder (Coherex Medical, Salt Lake City, UT) has a nitinol frame with an expanded polytetrafluoroethylene cover over foam backing with exposed and flexible fixation anchors (https://coherex.com/the-wavecrest-option/). The WaveCrest received CE approval in 2013, but has not yet received FDA approval.

The short design of this device makes it more feasible for proximal deployment in the LAA. The published data on this device (WAVECREST I) enrolled 73 patients with a mean $CHADS_2$ score of 2.5, prior stroke in 34%, and 49% with a contraindication to warfarin with procedure success in 96% (n = 70 of 73). Two patients developed tamponade during the implant procedure.[31]

LARIAT endocardial/epicardial suture delivery system

LARIAT (SentreHeart, Redwood City, CA) deployment involves a combined percutaneous endocardial and epicardial method of LAAC and may be advantageous for prevention of stroke and maintaining sinus rhythm (**Fig. 5**). Some potential advantages of the LARIAT closure system include suitability for large LAA orifice, lack of need for post-procedure anticoagulation, and potential elimination of electrical foci from and into the LAA. Patients with history of coronary artery bypass graft or pericarditis, however, may have adhesions in this space and therefore are not suitable for this procedure. Procedure safety remains a concern because cardiac tamponade and bleeding needing urgent surgery including one death have been reported.[32] Periprocedural use of colchicine has significantly decreased the risk of pericarditis and micropuncture needles for subxiphoid pericardial access have reduced the risk of cardiac perforation.[33] Studies have shown that successful occlusion of LAA with the LARIAT device has led to a decrease in AF burden in patients with proven LAA ectopy.[34] The currently enrolling aMAZE trial (ClinicalTrials.gov Identifier: NCT02513797) randomizes patients between pulmonary vein isolation alone versus a combined procedure of

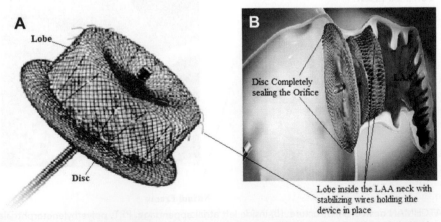

Fig. 4. Amulet. (*A*) Structure. (*B*) Inside LAA. (*Courtesy of* Abbott, Abbott Park, IL; with permission.)

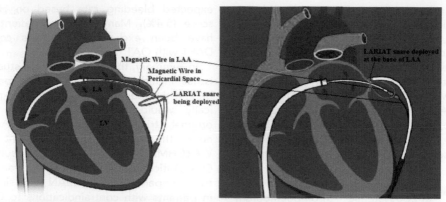

Fig. 5. LARIAT device system. LA, left atrium; LV, left ventricle. (*Courtesy of* SentreHeart, Redwood City, CA; with permission.)

pulmonary vein isolation and LAA ligation. It is powered to assess whether or not the addition of LAA ligation influences freedom from atrial arrhythmias post-procedure.[35]

PARADOX AND SOLUTION

PROTECT and PREVAIL were conducted in patients who were eligible for warfarin therapy.[20–23] However, the biggest unmet need for stroke prevention is in patients who are not candidates for OAC. LAAC offers an attractive alternative in such patients. Although there are no randomized data available in such patients and such trials are difficult to carry out, multiple nonrandomized studies have reported safety and efficacy in these patients.

ASAP Registry: Multicenter, Prospective, Observation Registry

The use of WATCHMAN device in patients with absolute contraindications to anticoagulation was evaluated in a prospective multicenter nonrandomized ASAP (ASA Plavix Feasibility Study with Watchman Left Atrial Appendage Closure Technology) study, which enrolled 150 patients with nonvalvular AF (CHADS$_2$ score $\geq$1) who had contraindication to anticoagulation being treated with WATCHMAN and 6 months of a thienopyridine (clopidogrel or ticlopidine) and lifelong aspirin.[36] Successful device implantation occurred in 95% and 8.7% (n = 13 of 150) of patients experienced procedure- or device-related serious adverse events (SAEs), including five pericardial effusions. During a mean duration of follow-up of 14.4 months, the primary efficacy outcome of all-cause stroke or systemic embolism occurred at a rate of 2.3% per year and ischemic stroke

occurred at a rate of 1.7% per year. This all-cause stroke rate was greater than 60% lower than predicted rates for CHADS$_2$-matched cohorts of individuals taking either aspirin (7.3%) or clopidogrel (5.0%) alone.

EWOLUTION Registry

The EWOLUTION registry is an observational, prospective, single-arm, multicenter study that was designed to collect real-world outcome data on the WATCHMAN device. A total of 1025 patients were enrolled at up to 47 medical centers in 13 countries (Europe, Russia, and in the Middle East).[37] Of these patients, 73.3% were deemed contraindicated to OAC therapy with history of prior hemorrhagic stroke and major bleeding in 15.1% and 31.3%, respectively. The average HAS-BLED score was 2.3 + 1.2 with HAS-BLED score of 3 or more in 40% of subjects. At baseline, only 31% of patients were on OAC therapy, 21% were on dual antiplatelet therapy (DAPT), 22% were on single antiplatelet therapy (APT), and 27% were not taking any form of anticoagulation. Patients had an average CHADS$_2$ score of 2.8 $\pm$ 1.3 and CHA$_2$DS$_2$-VASc score of 4.5 $\pm$ 1.6. An important finding from this registry was that after WATCHMAN implantation, only 27% of patients were on OAC therapy, 60% of subjects were on DAPT, 7% were on single APT, and 6% were not on any type of antiplatelet or anticoagulant therapy at all. However, during follow-up, discontinuation of clopidogrel and OAC therapy occurred and therefore 84% of patients ended up being on antiplatelet therapy (55% on single and 28% on dual) only and 9% receiving no therapy at all. The average time to discontinue DAPT was 6 months and 25% were changed to single agent within 3 months.

SAEs related to procedure and/or device (pericardial effusion, device embolization, major bleeding, vascular damage, air embolism, and reintervention for incomplete seal) occurred at a rate of 2.8% within the first week after implantation, much lower than any previous WATCHMAN LAAC studies (PROTECT-AF, 8.7%; CAP, 4.1%; PREVAIL, 4.2%). At 1-year follow-up, adequate sealing (<5 mm leak) was achieved in 99% of patients. Device thrombus was present in 3.7% (n = 28) of patients but with no correlation to post-procedure drug regimen. Combined annual ischemic/transient ischemic attack/systemic thromboembolism rate was 1.5% (85% risk reduction) with an annual ischemic stroke rate of 1.1% (84% risk reduction). Annual rate of bleeding (periprocedural and follow-up) was 2.6% translating into 48% risk reduction assuming that patients would be on VKA therapy otherwise. There was no difference in mortality, stroke, or bleeding rates between patients with or without contraindication to OAC therapy and also no correlation with type of anticoagulant used post-procedure.[38]

Canadian Multicenter Patient-Level Pooled Analysis for Safety and Efficacy of WATCHMAN Device Left Atrial Appendage Closure

This study included a total of 106 patients who underwent WATCHMAN device implantation from May 2013 to October 2015.[39] The mean CHADS$_2$ score was 2.8 ± 1.2, CHA$_2$DS$_2$Vasc score 4.7 ± 1.5, and HASBLED score 2 ± 1.2. Most of the subjects had history of prior bleeding (89.6%), with 82.1% having prior major bleeding and 28.3% having prior minor bleeding. Post-procedure therapy included DAPT in 73.8%, OAT in 20.4%, and aspirin alone in 2.9%. Most patients (11.7%) in the OAT group received NOAC alone for 6 weeks. The mean follow-up duration was 210.3 ± 182.2 days. The composite procedure major safety event rate was 1.9%, which included cardiovascular perforation with subsequent sepsis-related death at Day 5 and device embolization with percutaneous snare retrieval. The annual thromboembolic event rate at follow-up observed was 3.3% with a 66% and 59% relative reduction when compared with their event rate as per their CHADS2 and CHADSVasc score, respectively. Follow-up device surveillance revealed only one device-associated thrombus and no peridevice leak greater than 5 mm was reported. The observed major bleeding event rate during follow-up was 4.7%, which was similar to their expected bleeding rate based on HASBLED score (5.4%). Many of these patients would have been excluded from trials comparing DAPT with OAT (ACTIVE W).

In summary, these observational studies/registries include patients that could potentially benefit the most from LAAC and yet, paradoxically, would not have met criteria for the original trials randomizing to LAAC. Of note, the ASAP-TOO (Assessment of the WATCHMAN Device in Patients Unsuitable for Oral Anticoagulation) multicenter randomized trial comparing WATCHMAN with single APT in patients with contraindications to OAC will be launched soon but the results will not be available for at least 5 years. Although randomized data in this population are not yet available, available data from registries and nonrandomized studies suggest that LAAC can be performed safely in patients with contraindications to OAT with projected reduction in long-term thromboembolic event rates by approximately 60% to 70% with the WATCHMAN or ACP device.[28,36,40]

Left Atrial Appendage Closure with WATCHMAN Versus Novel Oral Anticoagulants

Koifman and colleagues[41] performed a meta-analysis, including 12 trials (randomized and nonrandomized) to compare the safety and efficacy of NOACs versus the LAAC with WATCHMAN device in patients with nonvalvular AF, in terms of hemorrhagic complications, stroke preventions, and all-cause mortality. The conclusion was that NOACs (OR, 0.46) and the WATCHMAN LAAC system (OR, 0.21) significantly decrease the risk of hemorrhagic stroke compared with warfarin. Both strategies were comparable and there was no difference between NOACs compared with the WATCHMAN device (OR, 1.25) when it came to major bleeding. Surprisingly, this meta-analysis showed that the LAAC with WATCHMAN did not significantly reduce the risk of hemorrhagic stroke compared with NOACS (OR, 0.44; 95% confidence interval, 0.09–2.14).[40] For all-cause mortality, there was a trend toward reduction for NOACs (OR, 0.66) and a weaker trend for WATCHMAN device (OR, 0.79) compared with warfarin.[21] Subgroup analysis including only randomized controlled trials suggested that NOACs led to a significant reduction in all-cause mortality (OR, 0.89) and hemorrhagic stroke (OR, 0.45) along with a trend toward reduction in total stroke (OR, 0.84) and major bleeding

(OR, 0.79), whereas WATCHMAN device was associated with only significant reduction in hemorrhagic stroke (OR, 0.19) and a trend toward reduction in all-cause mortality (OR, 0.68), when compared with warfarin. Subgroup analysis with data from randomized controlled trials only, comparing NOACs with WATCHMAN device, suggested no significant difference in regard to any outcome.[41]

INDICATIONS, PATIENT SELECTION, AND CURRENT GUIDELINES FOR LEFT ATRIAL APPENDAGE CLOSURE

The current American College of Cardiology/American Heart Association/Heart Rhythm Society guideline for the management of patients with AF does not include recommendations for the use of LAA occlusion devices because of the lack of adequate data and the absence of an FDA-approved LAAC device labeled for the indication of stroke prevention at the time of their development.[7] On March 13, 2015, the FDA issued an approval for the WATCHMAN device. The approval specified indications for use in patients with nonvalvular AF who are (1) at increased risk of stroke and systemic embolism based on CHADS$_2$ or CHA$_2$DS$_2$-VASc scores; (2) deemed by their physicians to be suitable for warfarin therapy; and (3) have an appropriate rationale to seek a nonpharmacologic alternative to warfarin, taking into account the safety and efficacy of the device compared with warfarin.[42]

American Heart Association/American Stroke Association guidelines state that closure of the LAA may be considered for high-risk patients with AF who are deemed unsuitable for anticoagulation if performed at a center with low rates of periprocedural complications and the patient can tolerate the risk of at least 45 days of postprocedural anticoagulation (class IIb; level of evidence B).[43]

European Society of Cardiology implemented a class IIB recommendation (level B) for LAAC for patients with nonvalvular AF who are either contraindicated or unsuitable for long-term OAT because of high bleeding risk (HASBLED score ≥3) or as an alternative treatment.[8]

According to the European Heart Rhythm Association and European Association of Percutaneous Cardiovascular Interventions, LAAC is recommended in patients with AF and indication for OAT for stroke/embolism prevention (with CHA$_2$DS$_2$-VASc score >1 point) and increased risk of bleeding (HAS-BLED score 3 points or

more), contraindications for OAT, or refusal of treatment with OAT.[44]

Many experts are concerned about the efficacy of LAAC compared with OAC therapy for preventing thromboembolic events, citing the randomized trials like PROTECT AF/PREVAIL as evidence. However, it is important to understand the paradox between the available randomized data and the unmet clinical need for stroke prevention being promised by LAAC, as described previously. Regardless of the paradox the results from these trials were promising for LAAC, because it significantly reduced the incidence of hemorrhagic events. Strategies like shortened DAPT, low-dose NOACs, or single antiplatelet courses post-procedure may be considered in LAAC patients with high bleeding risk deemed not suitable for OAC therapy. Based on the plentiful data from different registries about successful use of LAAC in patients with contraindication to anticoagulation and also on the efficacy and safety of different antithrombotic protocols post-procedure, the following group of patients would likely benefit from LAAC (**Fig. 6**):

1. Thrombocytopenia or known coagulation defect associated with bleeding.
2. Recurrent gastrointestinal bleeding.
3. Prior severe bleeding, including ICH. Recurrent ICH has devastating consequences for a patient and therefore most of these patients are not on any OAC therapy. A troubling finding is that the rate of ischemic events also is increased in patients with prior history of ICH,[45] making it an important indication for LAAC. A recent prospective multicenter ACP registry suggested that LAAC was a safe procedure with similar procedure outcomes in patients with and without previous ICH and was associated with reduced thromboembolic and significantly reduced hemorrhagic events compared with expected rates as per CHA$_2$DS$_2$-VASc and HASBLED score, respectively. The use of less intensive antithrombotic therapy after LAAC in patients with previous ICH was not associated with increase in the frequency of device thrombosis or peridevice leaks.[28]
4. Combined use of DAPT and anticoagulant therapy. The bleeding risk is substantial in patients on "triple therapy" (4%–12% at 1 year).[46] In these patients, even without a prior bleeding event, the benefit/risk ratio may favor LAAC over triple therapy.
5. Poor compliance with anticoagulant therapy.

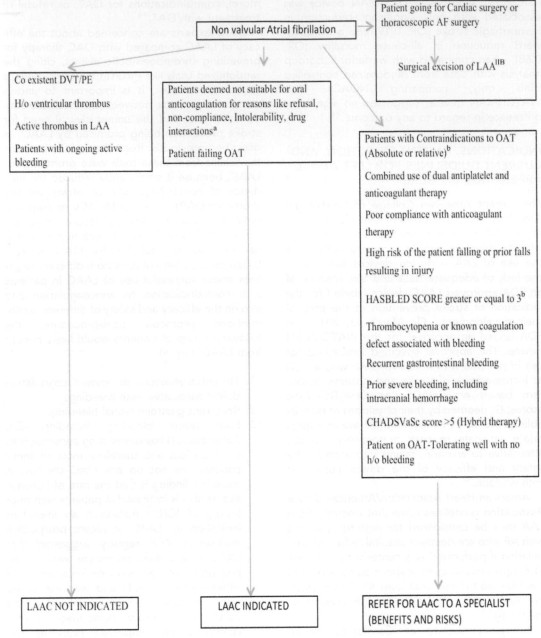

Fig. 6. Flow chart depicting the patient selection (indications) for LAAC. [IIB] European Society of Cardiology; American Heart Association/American College of Cardiology recommendation. [a] FDA guideline for LAAC. [b] European Society of Cardiology class IIb recommendation. DVT, deep venous thrombosis; PE, pulmonary embolism.

6. High risk of the patient falling or prior falls resulting in injury.
7. Failed OAC therapy in preventing thromboembolic phenomenon.
8. HASBLED SCORE ≥3.
9. Other patients with an absolute contraindication to anticoagulation: a multicenter prospective nonrandomized

trial in Canada in patients with nonvalvular AF and absolute contraindications to OAC (ICH, 34.6%; gastrointestinal bleeding, 23.1%; or spontaneous hematoma of abdominal muscles, 13.5%) was carried out by Urena and colleagues[40] in which LAAC with ACP was followed by DAPT (1–3 months) and then APT. There was a low rate of embolic and bleeding events after a mean follow-up of 20 months with a procedure success rate of 98.1%. There were no cases of device thrombosis or periprocedural stroke.

10. As an alternative to OAC therapy in patients on an OAC regimen with no contraindication to LAAC. The randomized trials showing noninferiority of LAAC versus Warfarin were carried out on such patients. The need for monitoring of effect and narrow therapeutic window of warfarin and the lack of an FDA-approved antidote to factor Xa inhibitors and associated cost issues with NOACs[47,48] may lead patients and providers to consider LAAC as an alternative to OAC. Studies comparing the safety, efficacy, and cost effectiveness of LAAC to NOACs are needed.

The following patient data are helpful in patient selection for LAAC:

- Risk for stroke: CHA_2DS_2-VASc SCORE
- Risk for bleeding: HASBLED score
- Prior experience with OAC and antithrombotic therapy
- Contraindications to OAC or antithrombotic therapy, absolute and relative
- Cardiac structure and function including LAA anatomy
- Feasibility of percutaneous approach for LAA occlusion

Patient selection for this procedure continues to be on a case-by-case basis and shared decision making is critical.[49]

Potential Benefits and Areas for Future Investigation

Left atrial appendage exclusion (LARIAT) as an adjunct to atrial fibrillation ablation

It is well known that LAA has a role in pathophysiology of AF in some patients[50] explaining the outcome of decreased AF burden in patients who underwent LARIAT exclusion.[34] The currently enrolling aMAZE trial will shed more light on the prospects of LARIAT in this direction.

Patients with end-stage renal disease and advanced chronic kidney disease

These patients have increased risk of thromboembolic and bleeding events.[51,52] The evidence does not suggest a clear benefit of OAC in these patients and many were excluded from the NOAC trials. LAAC may be a reasonable alternative to OAC in this population and further studies are needed.

Patients with bleeding diatheses

Patients with bleeding diatheses who can tolerate antiplatelet agents but not OAC represent another group of patients where LAAC might offer a reasonable option for prevention of thromboembolic phenomenon. There is plenty of evidence from observational studies, such as the Canadian multicenter trial, regarding the efficacy of different antithrombotic protocols following LAAC. Prospective, randomized studies would provide more definitive conclusions.

Patients with high CHA_2DS_2-VASc score (5 or more)

ROCKET AF trial showed that patients with CHA_2DS_2-VASc score of 5 or more had a 2-year event rate in excess of five events per 100 patient-years despite anticoagulation.[52] Such patients with high "residual risk" might potentially benefit from hybrid therapy in which indefinite OAC (with low-dose NOAC) is combined with LAAC.

Patients with symptomatic atrial fibrillation undergoing ablation

The concept of combing these two procedures in a single setting is another exciting perspective that needs further study. Despite the risk of long-term recurrence, catheter ablation remains more effective than antiarrhythmic drugs in terms of freedom of AF and/or its symptoms.[53,54] Combining ablation with LAAC might result in further symptomatic improvement and patient satisfaction, lower the LAA-associated thromboembolic risk, and eliminate the need for long-term OAC therapy. There may be benefits with some LAAC techniques toward rhythm control. A report on 30 patients showed that a combined procedure is feasible and safe with a median additional procedure time of only 38 minutes provided there were no LAAC-associated complications.[55] In another study, Arash Alipour and colleagues[56] showed that after a median follow-up of around 3 years, 78% (39 or 50) of patients with a mean CHADS2 score of 2.5 had their OAC discontinued during their follow-up. The rate of ischemic stroke was 1.7% in this patient population, which was lower than the expected rate for their $CHADS_2$ score (6.5%). There was no compromise on the success rate of catheter ablation, as evident in the literature. Another study showed similar satisfactory results for freedom from AF and OAC therapy but a higher rate of procedure-related complications (8.6% cardiac tamponade).[57]

Cost-effectiveness of left atrial appendage closure

This procedure has also proven to be cost effective when compared with aspirin after 5 years, warfarin after 7 years, and the NOACs after 5 to 7 years and is expected to stay like that for the next two decades.[58,59] Given the significant decrease in procedure-related complications with time, higher operator experience, and advancement in device technology, LAAC is becoming a safer procedure and may offer an alternative first-line treatment of stroke prevention in patients with nonvalvular AF.

Patients Who Should Not Undergo Left Atrial Appendage Closure

Patients who are already on an OAT therapy (NOAC or warfarin) for nonvalvular AF with no complications or side effects and are amenable to continued therapy are not candidates for LAAC. Presently there is not sufficient evidence to support switching these patients from OAC therapy to LAAC. Further study is needed.

Patients with valvular AF should not undergo LAAC. There is insufficient evidence regarding the role of LAAC in this patient population.

Patients who have indications for OAC therapy other than valvular AF (ie, mechanical valve, venous thromboembolism, left ventricular thrombus) also should not undergo LAAC.

Although there are case reports where LAAC was successfully used in patients with an active clot in LAA using a triguard embolic protection system,[60] routine use of LAAC in patients with an active or suspected LAA thrombus is not presently advised. Further investigation is warranted.

Patients with ongoing, active bleeding are also not candidates for LAAC because intraprocedural anticoagulation is currently required for LAAC.

Post left atrial appendage closure challenges

1. Risk of bleeding with antithrombotic therapy used after LAAC: Patients who undergo LAAC still require long-term antiplatelet therapies and therefore are exposed to continued bleeding risk, which is comparable with risk with OAC as reported in some studies. For example, AVERROES trial has actually shown that major bleeding was not significantly different between APIXABAN and the aspirin group (1.4 vs 1.2% per year; hazard ratio, 1.13; 95% confidence interval, 0.74–1.75; P = .57). Similarly, there was no difference in intracranial bleeding.[9]

2. LAA leak: can be peridevice (with endocardial devices, such as WATCHMAN or ACP) or a central "gunny sack" leak as observed with the LARIAT suture exclusion.[61] A Doppler flow jet less than 5 mm is not considered clinically significant and may resolve on follow-up imaging. Overall prevalence of leaks associated with WATCHMAN device is high (30%-45% at 1-year follow-up). With LARIAT, the prevalence of leaks is low compared with endocardial devices (20% at 1-year follow-up)[62] with most ranging from 1 to 3 mm and are easy to close with ACP plugs unlike peridevice leaks. Post hoc analysis of the PROTECT AF data did not suggest any increased risk of stroke in patients with minor or major leaks compared with patients with no leak.[63] In another multicenter observational study, 3 patients out of 259 had a stroke after LARIAT LAA exclusion and all three had documented complete closure of the LAA.[61] Secondary closure of leaks with the AMPLATZER occluder device has been reported in LARIAT- and WATCHMAN-treated patients[64,65] and may be a viable option in some patients. A fluid bolus before implant, by enlarging LAA dimensions, may improve the fitting of the device into LAA and thereby lower the risk of LAA leak.[66] Long-term data on the future risk of systemic thromboembolism are largely unknown.

3. Device-associated thrombus formation. In the PROTECT AF trial, follow-up with TEE revealed 4.2% of successfully implanted devices had thrombus formation on them. The rate of stroke in these patients was low at 0.3 events per 100 patient-years.[67] However, the current guidelines recommend continuation of anticoagulation until thrombus resolves.[27]

4. In patients with AF, thromboembolic phenomenon from LAA is not the only mechanism for stroke. AF itself is associated with a hypercoagulable state.[68,69] Available data from studies have shown that 45% of strokes occur without any AF event within the last 1 month of the stroke.[70]

REFERRAL PATHWAY

There are many stroke prevention options for patients with AF, ranging from pharmacologic to mechanical measures. It is of high importance to have a proper referral system in place for

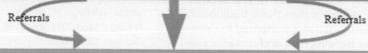

EDUCATION
- Educate Patients and family about the disease and possible treatment options available
- Educate PCP's, NP's, about the new interventions available for stroke prevention in high risk Atrial fibrillation patients
- Educate about LAAC procedure and it's potential risks and benefits via Brochures, Website Info
- Explain the process from screening→procedure→ follow up

Referrals   Referrals

SCREENING
- Pre Screening can be done over Phone by Trained Nurse Coordinators
- Secure Insurance Pre-Authorization for the procedure
- Schedule an office visit to review Medical records-make sure patient is an appropriate candidate for LAAC procedure.
- Review Previous TEE/TTE/CT Imaging. Schedule for new TEE if none available to ensure patient is a good candidate (size, thrombus, etc.)

SCHEDULING
- Schedule pre-procedure diagnostic studies, labs, echo, etc
- Schedule procedure date for lab time, implanter, anesthesia, TEE physician, patient, company representative (LAAC team)

PROCEDURE
- Ensure that patient has followed the pre-procedure instructions
- Ensure that all the key players involved in the procedure are present (LAAC team)
- Discharge patients on appropriate antithrombotic protocol
- Schedule post-procedure follow-up office visit, labs and TEE at the time of discharge
- Post procedure- Ensure that patient and family understand post procedure instructions (medication, follow up TEE date, etc.)

FOLLOW UP
- 1ST follow up office visit- as per the hospital protocol
- First follow up TEE at 45 d post procedure to assess for residual leaks and thrombus formation. Modify the antithrombotic regimen as per the findings.
- 6 mo follow up office visit-Usually all the Antithrombotic regimen is discontinued at this stage except for ASA
- 2nd follow up TEE may be performed at 1 y post procedure to assess for thrombus formation on the device while on ASA

Fig. 7. Outline of the proposed referral system for LAAC. ASA, acetylsalicylic acid; CT, computed tomography; TTE, transthoracic echocardiography.

patients that may benefit from LAAC. A strategic referral system is needed and awareness of LAAC by providers caring for patients with non-valvular AF. The goal of this referral system is timely referral and a smooth transition of care for appropriate patients. Our proposed referral is demonstrated in **Fig. 7.**

SUMMARY

LAAC offers an elegant and feasible option for prevention of thromboembolism in patients with nonvalvular AF, particularly in those with a rational reason to avoid OAC. Patient selection remains a challenge because of the paradox between the available randomized data on this intervention and the actual patient cohort most in need of this procedure. Fortunately, observational data support extension of LAAC to patients most in need with excellent results thus far. Its use must continue to be tailored to the individual patient, occasionally with less vigorous post-procedure antithrombotic regimens than those traditionally used. Further investigation is warranted to determine the relative benefits, risks, and cost effectiveness of LAAC as compared with NOAC in patients not intolerant, refusing, or with a contraindication to OAC. Furthermore, the optimal antithrombotic regimen post-procedure has yet to be determined. Comparative data between the various LAAC devices are forthcoming and will be insightful in tailoring this promising therapy to individual patients.

REFERENCES

1. Lip GYH, Brechin CM, Lane DA. The global burden of atrial fibrillation and stroke: a systematic review of the epidemiology of atrial fibrillation in regions outside North America and Europe. Chest 2012; 142(6):1489–98.

2. Ball J, Carrington MJ, McMurray JJ, et al. Atrial fibrillation: profile and burden of an evolving epidemic in the 21st century. Int J Cardiol 2013; 167(5):1807–24.

3. Chugh SS, Havmoeller R, Narayanan K, et al. Worldwide epidemiology of atrial fibrillation: a Global Burden of Disease 2010 study. Circulation 2014;129(8):837–47.

4. Wolf PA, Abbott RD, Kannel WB. Atrial fibrillation as an independent risk factor for stroke: the Framingham Study. Stroke 1991;22(8):983–8.

5. Go AS, Hylek EM, Phillips KA, et al. Prevalence of diagnosed atrial fibrillation in adults: national implications for rhythm management and stroke prevention: the AnTicoagulation and Risk Factors in Atrial Fibrillation (ATRIA) Study. JAMA 2001;285(18): 2370–5.

6. Blackshear JL, Odell JA. Appendage obliteration to reduce stroke in cardiac surgical patients with atrial fibrillation. Ann Thorac Surg 1996;61(2):755–9.

7. January CT, Wann LS, Alpert JS, et al. 2014 AHA/ACC/HRS guideline for the management of patients with atrial fibrillation: a report of the American College of Cardiology/American Heart Association Task Force on Practice Guidelines and the Heart Rhythm Society. J Am Coll Cardiol 2014;64(21):e1–76.

8. Kirchhof P, Benussi S, Kotecha D, et al. 2016 ESC Guidelines for the management of atrial fibrillation developed in collaboration with EACTS. Eur Heart J 2016;37(38):2893–962.

9. Connolly SJ, Eikelboom J, Joyner C, et al. Apixaban in patients with atrial fibrillation. N Engl J Med 2011;364(9):806–17.

10. Connolly SJ, Ezekowitz MD, Yusuf S, et al. Dabigatran versus warfarin in patients with atrial fibrillation. N Engl J Med 2009;361(12):1139–51.

11. Patel MR, Mahaffey KW, Garg J, et al. Rivaroxaban versus warfarin in nonvalvular atrial fibrillation. N Engl J Med 2011;365(10):883–91.

12. Granger CB, Alexander JH, McMurray JJ, et al. Apixaban versus warfarin in patients with atrial fibrillation. N Engl J Med 2011;365(11):981–92.

13. Turagam MK, Parikh V, Afzal MR, et al. Replacing warfarin with a novel oral anticoagulant: risk of recurrent bleeding and stroke in patients with warfarin ineligible or failure in patients with atrial fibrillation (The ROAR study). J Cardiovasc Electrophysiol 2017;28(8):853–61.

14. Kachroo S, Hamilton M, Liu X, et al. Oral anticoagulant discontinuation in patients with nonvalvular atrial fibrillation. Am J Manag Care 2016;22(1): e1–8.

15. Tsai YC, Phan K, Munkholm-Larsen S, et al. Surgical left atrial appendage occlusion during cardiac surgery for patients with atrial fibrillation: a meta-analysis. Eur J Cardiothorac Surg 2015;47(5):847–54.

16. January CT, Wann LS, Alpert JS, et al. 2014 AHA/ACC/HRS guideline for the management of patients with atrial fibrillation: executive summary: a report of the American College of Cardiology/American Heart Association Task Force on practice guidelines and the Heart Rhythm Society. Circulation 2014;130(23):2071–104.

17. Kanderian AS, Gillinov AM, Pettersson GB, et al. Success of surgical left atrial appendage closure: assessment by transesophageal echocardiography. J Am Coll Cardiol 2008;52(11):924–9.

18. Cullen MW, Stulak JM, Li Z, et al. Left atrial appendage patency at cardioversion after surgical left atrial appendage intervention. Ann Thorac Surg 2016;101(2):675–81.

19. Ailawadi G, Gerdisch MW, Harvey RL, et al. Exclusion of the left atrial appendage with a novel device: early results of a multicenter trial. J Thorac Cardiovasc Surg 2011;142(5):1002–9, 1009.e1.

20. Holmes DR, Reddy VY, Turi ZG, et al. Percutaneous closure of the left atrial appendage versus warfarin therapy for prevention of stroke in patients with atrial fibrillation: a randomised non-inferiority trial. Lancet 2009;374(9689):534–42.

21. Reddy VY, Doshi SK, Sievert H, et al. Percutaneous left atrial appendage closure for stroke prophylaxis in patients with atrial fibrillation: 2.3-year follow-up of the PROTECT AF (Watchman Left Atrial Appendage System for Embolic Protection in Patients with Atrial Fibrillation) Trial. Circulation 2013;127(6):720–9.

22. Holmes DR Jr, Kar S, Price MJ, et al. Prospective randomized evaluation of the Watchman left atrial appendage closure device in patients with atrial fibrillation versus long-term warfarin therapy: the PREVAIL trial. J Am Coll Cardiol 2014;64(1):1–12.

23. Holmes DR Jr, Doshi SK, Kar S, et al. Left atrial appendage closure as an alternative to warfarin for stroke prevention in atrial fibrillation: a patient-level meta-analysis. J Am Coll Cardiol 2015;65(24):2614–23.

24. Enomoto Y, Gadiyaram VK, Gianni C, et al. Use of non-warfarin oral anticoagulants instead of warfarin during left atrial appendage closure with the Watchman device. Heart Rhythm 2017;14(1):19–24.

25. Park JW, Bethencourt A, Sievert H, et al. Left atrial appendage closure with Amplatzer cardiac plug in atrial fibrillation: initial European experience. Catheter Cardiovasc Interv 2011;77(5):700–6.

26. Freixa X, Chan JL, Tzikas A, et al. The Amplatzer Cardiac Plug 2 for left atrial appendage occlusion: novel features and first-in-man experience. EuroIntervention 2013;8(9):1094–8.

27. Meier B, Blaauw Y, Khattab AA, et al. EHRA/EAPCI expert consensus statement on catheter-based left atrial appendage occlusion. Europace 2014;16(10):1397–416.

28. Tzikas A, Shakir S, Gafoor S, et al. Left atrial appendage occlusion for stroke prevention in atrial fibrillation: multicentre experience with the AMPLATZER Cardiac Plug. EuroIntervention 2016;11(10):1170–9.

29. Abualsaud A, Freixa X, Tzikas A, et al. Side-by-side comparison of LAA occlusion performance with the Amplatzer cardiac plug and Amplatzer amulet. J Invasive Cardiol 2016;28(1):34–8.

30. Freixa X, Abualsaud A, Chan J, et al. Left atrial appendage occlusion: initial experience with the Amplatzer Amulet. Int J Cardiol 2014;174(3):492–6.

31. Reddy VY, Franzen O, Worthley S, et al. Clinical experience with the WaveCrest LA appendage occlusion device for stroke prevention in AF: acute results of the WAVECREST I trial. Heart Rhythm Society 35th Annual scientific session. San Francisco (CA), May 7–10, 2014. p. P001-112.

32. Chatterjee S, Herrmann HC, Wilensky RL, et al. Safety and procedural success of left atrial appendage exclusion with the lariat device: a systematic review of published reports and analytic review of the FDA MAUDE database. JAMA Intern Med 2015;175(7):1104–9.

33. Lakkireddy D, Afzal MR, Lee RJ, et al. Short and long-term outcomes of percutaneous left atrial appendage suture ligation: results from a US multicenter evaluation. Heart Rhythm 2016;13(5):1030–6.

34. Afzal MR, Kanmanthareddy A, Earnest M, et al. Impact of left atrial appendage exclusion using an epicardial ligation system (LARIAT) on atrial fibrillation burden in patients with cardiac implantable electronic devices. Heart Rhythm 2015;12(1):52–9.

35. Lee RJ, Lakkireddy D, Mittal S, et al. Percutaneous alternative to the Maze procedure for the treatment of persistent or long-standing persistent atrial fibrillation (aMAZE trial): rationale and design. Am Heart J 2015;170(6):1184–94.

36. Reddy VY, Mobius-Winkler S, Miller MA, et al. Left atrial appendage closure with the Watchman device in patients with a contraindication for oral anticoagulation: the ASAP study (ASA Plavix feasibility study with Watchman left atrial appendage closure technology). J Am Coll Cardiol 2013;61(25):2551–6.

37. Boersma LV, Schmidt B, Betts TR, et al. Implant success and safety of left atrial appendage closure with the WATCHMAN device: peri-procedural outcomes from the EWOLUTION registry. Eur Heart J 2016;37(31):2465–74.

38. Boersma LV, Ince H, Kische S, et al. Efficacy and safety of left atrial appendage closure with WATCHMAN in patients with or without contraindication to oral anticoagulation: 1-year follow-up outcome data of the EWOLUTION trial. Heart Rhythm 2017;14(9):1302–8.

39. Saw J, Fahmy P, Azzalini L, et al. Early Canadian multicenter experience with WATCHMAN for percutaneous left atrial appendage closure. J Cardiovasc Electrophysiol 2017;28(4):396–401.

40. Urena M, Rodes-Cabau J, Freixa X, et al. Percutaneous left atrial appendage closure with the AMPLATZER cardiac plug device in patients with nonvalvular atrial fibrillation and contraindications to anticoagulation therapy. J Am Coll Cardiol 2013;62(2):96–102.

41. Koifman E, Lipinski MJ, Escarcega RO, et al. Comparison of Watchman device with new oral anticoagulants in patients with atrial fibrillation: a network meta-analysis. Int J Cardiol 2016;205:17–22.

42. FDA Approval for WATCHMAN Device. Available at: http://www.accessdata.fda.gov/cdrh_docs/pdf13/P130013a.pdf. Accessed March 24, 2015.

43. Meschia JF, Bushnell C, Boden-Albala B, et al. Guidelines for the primary prevention of stroke: a statement for healthcare professionals from the American Heart Association/American Stroke Association. Stroke 2014;45(12):3754–832.

44. Meier B, Blaauw Y, Khattab AA, et al. EHRA/EAPCI expert consensus statement on catheter-based left atrial appendage occlusion. EuroIntervention 2015;10(9):1109–25.

45. Lerario MP, Gialdini G, Lapidus DM, et al. Risk of ischemic stroke after intracranial hemorrhage in patients with atrial fibrillation. PLoS One 2015;10(12):e0145579.

46. Faxon DP, Eikelboom JW, Berger PB, et al. Antithrombotic therapy in patients with atrial fibrillation undergoing coronary stenting: a North American perspective: executive summary. Circ Cardiovasc Interv 2011;4(5):522–34.

47. Cowell RP. Direct oral anticoagulants: integration into clinical practice. Postgrad Med J 2014; 90(1067):529–39.

48. Gallego P, Roldan V, Lip GY. Novel oral anticoagulants in cardiovascular disease. J Cardiovasc Pharmacol Ther 2014;19(1):34–44.

49. Barry MJ, Edgman-Levitan S. Shared decision making: pinnacle of patient-centered care. N Engl J Med 2012;366(9):780–1.

50. Di Biase L, Burkhardt JD, Mohanty P, et al. Left atrial appendage: an underrecognized trigger site of atrial fibrillation. Circulation 2010;122(2): 109–18.

51. Shah M, Avgil Tsadok M, Jackevicius CA, et al. Warfarin use and the risk for stroke and bleeding in patients with atrial fibrillation undergoing dialysis. Circulation 2014;129(11): 1196–203.

52. Piccini JP, Stevens SR, Chang Y, et al. Renal dysfunction as a predictor of stroke and systemic embolism in patients with nonvalvular atrial fibrillation: validation of the R(2)CHADS(2) index in the ROCKET AF (Rivaroxaban Once-daily, oral, direct factor Xa inhibition Compared with vitamin K antagonism for prevention of stroke and Embolism Trial in Atrial Fibrillation) and ATRIA (AnTicoagulation and Risk factors In Atrial fibrillation) study cohorts. Circulation 2013;127(2):224–32.

53. Pappone C, Augello G, Sala S, et al. A randomized trial of circumferential pulmonary vein ablation versus antiarrhythmic drug therapy in paroxysmal atrial fibrillation: the APAF Study. J Am Coll Cardiol 2006;48(11):2340–7.

54. Stabile G, Bertaglia E, Senatore G, et al. Catheter ablation treatment in patients with drug-refractory atrial fibrillation: a prospective, multi-centre, randomized, controlled study (catheter ablation for the cure of atrial fibrillation study). Eur Heart J 2006;27(2):216–21.

55. Swaans MJ, Post MC, Rensing BJ, et al. Ablation for atrial fibrillation in combination with left atrial appendage closure: first results of a feasibility study. J Am Heart Assoc 2012;1(5):e002212.

56. Alipour A, Swaans MJ, van Dijk VF, et al. Ablation for atrial fibrillation combined with left atrial appendage closure. JACC: Clinical Electrophysiology 2015;1(6):486–95.

57. Calvo N, Salterain N, Arguedas H, et al. Combined catheter ablation and left atrial appendage closure as a hybrid procedure for the treatment of atrial fibrillation. Europace 2015;17(10):1533–40.

58. Reddy VY, Akehurst RL, Armstrong SO, et al. Cost effectiveness of left atrial appendage closure with the Watchman device for atrial fibrillation patients with absolute contraindications to warfarin. Europace 2016;18(7):979–86.

59. Reddy VY, Akehurst RL, Armstrong SO, et al. Time to cost-effectiveness following stroke reduction strategies in AF: warfarin versus NOACs versus LAA closure. J Am Coll Cardiol 2015;66(24): 2728–39.

60. Del Furia F, Ancona MB, Giannini F, et al. First-in-man percutaneous LAA closure with an Amplatzer amulet and TriGuard embolic protection device in a patient with LAA thrombus. J Invasive Cardiol 2017;29(4):E51–2.

61. Pillarisetti J, Reddy YM, Gunda S, et al. Endocardial (Watchman) vs epicardial (Lariat) left atrial appendage exclusion devices: understanding the differences in the location and type of leaks and their clinical implications. Heart Rhythm 2015; 12(7):1501–7.

62. Gianni C, Di Biase L, Trivedi C, et al. Clinical implications of leaks following left atrial appendage ligation with the LARIAT device. JACC Cardiovasc Interv 2016;9(10):1051–7.

63. Viles-Gonzalez JF, Kar S, Douglas P, et al. The clinical impact of incomplete left atrial appendage closure with the Watchman device in patients with atrial fibrillation: a PROTECT AF (percutaneous closure of the left atrial appendage versus warfarin therapy for prevention of stroke in patients with atrial fibrillation) substudy. J Am Coll Cardiol 2012;59(10):923–9.

64. Pillai AM, Kanmanthareddy A, Earnest M, et al. Initial experience with post Lariat left atrial appendage leak closure with Amplatzer septal occluder device and repeat Lariat application. Heart Rhythm 2014;11(11):1877–83.

65. Lam SC, Bertog S, Sievert H. Incomplete left atrial appendage occlusion and thrombus formation after Watchman implantation treated with anticoagulation followed by further transcatheter closure with a second-generation Amplatzer Cardiac Plug (Amulet device). Catheter Cardiovasc Interv 2015; 85(2):321–7.

66. Spencer RJ, DeJong P, Fahmy P, et al. Changes in left atrial appendage dimensions following volume loading during percutaneous left atrial appendage closure. JACC Cardiovasc Interv 2015; 8(15):1935–41.

67. Reddy VY, Holmes D, Doshi SK, et al. Safety of percutaneous left atrial appendage closure: results from the Watchman left atrial appendage system for embolic protection in patients with AF

(PROTECT AF) clinical trial and the Continued Access Registry. Circulation 2011;123(4):417–24.

68. Uno M, Tsuji H, Sawada S, et al. (FPA) levels in atrial fibrillation and the effects of heparin administration. Jpn Circ J 1988;52(1):9–12.

69. Mitusch R, Siemens HJ, Garbe M, et al. Detection of a hypercoagulable state in nonvalvular atrial fibrillation and the effect of anticoagulant therapy. Thromb Haemost 1996;75(2):219–23.

70. Glotzer TV, Daoud EG, Wyse DG, et al. The relationship between daily atrial tachyarrhythmia burden from implantable device diagnostics and stroke risk: the TRENDS study. Circ Arrhythm Electrophysiol 2009;2(5):474–80.

Anatomy and Physiologic Roles of the Left Atrial Appendage
Implications for Endocardial and Epicardial Device Closure

Nicholas Y. Tan, MD, MS[a], Omar Z. Yasin, MD, MS[a],
Alan Sugrue, MB, BCh, BAO[b], Abdallah El Sabbagh, MD[b],
Thomas A. Foley, MD[b], Samuel J. Asirvatham, MD[b],*

KEYWORDS

- Left atrial appendage anatomy • Percutaneous device closure • Atrial fibrillation
- Watchman device • Amplatzer cardiac plug • Lariat approach

KEY POINTS

- The left atrial appendage is a complex cardiac structure that harbors many variations in size, morphology, and position.
- Subtle differences in left atrial appendage anatomy can have a significant impact on the outcomes of current exclusion device procedures (Watchman, Amplatzer Cardiac Plug, and Lariat).
- It is imperative for the invasive cardiologist to consider these anatomic factors when selecting a suitable left atrial appendage exclusion approach for individual patients.

INTRODUCTION

The left atrial appendage (LAA) is a muscular, tubular structure that is an outpouching from the left atrium (LA). Similar to its namesake in the large intestine, it was previously regarded as a vestigial aspect of cardiac anatomy with little clinical consequence. However, in the 1950s, the LAA was discovered to play a key role in thrombus formation and cerebrovascular accidents, particularly in the setting of atrial fibrillation (AF).[1] Given that more than 90% of thrombi originate from the LAA, there has been intense interest in developing devices that exclude it and thereby reduce the risk of thromboembolism.[1]

At present, there are 3 LAA exclusion procedures used or tested across the United States and Europe: the Watchman (Atritech Inc, Plymouth, MI)[2,3]; the Amplatzer Cardiac Plug (ACP)[4] (St. Jude Medical, MI) and its second-generation counterpart the Amulet[5,6]; and the Lariat (SentreHEART Inc, Redwood City, CA) approach.[7] Although the overall concept of LAA exclusion is seemingly straightforward, subtle nuances in LAA anatomy and its neighboring entities can have a significant impact on the feasibility and success of these techniques.[8–15] As devices and procedures for LAA exclusion continue to evolve, it becomes increasingly important for both general and interventional cardiologists to be armed with a working

---

Disclosure Statement: All authors declare that they have no relevant financial interests to disclose.

[a] Department of Internal Medicine, Mayo Clinic Rochester, 200 1st Street Southwest, Rochester, MN 55905, USA;
[b] Department of Cardiovascular Diseases, Mayo Clinic Rochester, 200 1st Street Southwest, Rochester, MN 55905, USA
* Corresponding author.
E-mail address: asirvatham.samuel@mayo.edu

Intervent Cardiol Clin 7 (2018) 185–199
https://doi.org/10.1016/j.iccl.2017.12.001
2211-7458/18/© 2017 Elsevier Inc. All rights reserved.

knowledge of the LAA's development, anatomic variations, and spatial relationships so as to optimize patient care in terms of cerebrovascular accident risk reduction. With this in mind, we aim to describe the anatomy of the LAA and its implications on epicardial or endocardial device closure. We highlight the relevant aspects of LAA embryology, internal and external anatomy, as well as relationships with surrounding structures. We also review current options for LAA exclusion and the key anatomic considerations that relate to their suitability.

DEVELOPMENTAL ANATOMY

There are 5 major steps involved in the formation of the LAA. Gastrulation occurs at the third week of gestation, leading to the creation of the 3 embryonic layers (the ectoderm, mesoderm, and endoderm).[16] An inverted Y-shaped primary endocardial tube is formed by 2 populations of mesodermal cells arising from the crescent formation and secondary heart field (Fig. 1).[16,17] Elongation and looping of the endocardial tube then take place on day 25, bringing its caudal and cranial ends in close proximity.[16,17] At this time, several key structures of the future heart can be delineated; these include the conotruncus, primary ventricle, atrioventricular canal, sinus venosus, and primary atrium.[18]

The superolateral walls of the primary atrium begin "ballooning" outward, giving rise to the prototypical right and left atria, with the latter structure receiving a relatively greater contribution.[16,19,20] In a process called intussusception, cells from the sinus venosus are incorporated into the developing right atrium, whereas the pulmonary veins contribute to the dorsal wall

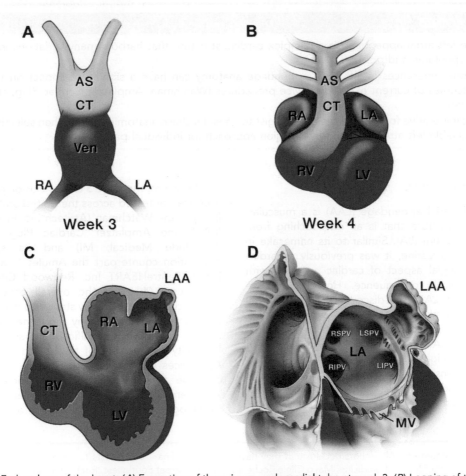

Fig. 1. Embryology of the heart. (A) Formation of the primary endocardial tube at week 3. (B) Looping of the tube at week 4. (C) Ballooning of the atria and formation of the LAA. (D) LA and LAA in the adult human heart. AS, aortic sac; CT, conotruncus; LA, left atrium; LAA, left atrial appendage; LIPV, left inferior pulmonary vein; LSPV, left superior pulmonary vein; LV, left ventricle; RA, right atrium; RIPV, right inferior pulmonary vein; RSPV, right superior pulmonary vein; RV, right ventricle; Ven, primary ventricle. (Courtesy of Mayo Foundation for Medical Education and Research, Rochester, MI; with permission.)

of the LA.[16,18,20] The outpouching along the superolateral aspect of the LA wall then persists as the LAA.[19,21] By the fifth week of gestation, the original cardiac mesoderm differentiates into muscle tissue, leading to trabeculations in parts of the LA as well as the LAA.[18,22]

ANATOMIC SHAPES AND VARIANTS
General Anatomic Description
The LAA is a complex and heterogeneous structure, but its essential components can be broken down into an ostium, neck, and body. The ostium connects the LA to the LAA and tends to run at an oblique angle to the mitral annulus. The superior and posterior borders of the ostium are generally well-demarcated by a ridgelike fold (Fig. 2) that separates the os from the left superior pulmonary vein (LSPV), whereas the anterior and inferior borders are less obviously defined.[14] This ridge, which corresponds epicardially with the ligament of Marshall, has been studied in detail[23–25] and a classification has been proposed: type A, in which the ridge extends from the superior portion of the LSPV orifice to the inferior portion of the left inferior pulmonary vein; and type B, where the ridge extends from the superior portion of the LSPV orifice to the left superior and inferior intervenous saddle.[26] The ostium is often at the same level as the LSPV (60%–65% of individuals), but it can also be superior to it (25%–30%) or inferior (10%–15%). The neck is typically the narrowest

part of the LAA and this region usually overlies the course of the left circumflex artery (LCX).[27] There is wide anatomic variation in the distance between the ostium and the neck. The body of the LAA is often multilobed (range, 1–4), usually containing 2 lobes per person in 54% of the population and 3 lobes in 23%.[28] The body of the LAA is trabeculated with pectinate muscles and in 28% these can be found extending inferiorly from the appendage to the vestibule of the mitral valve.[25] The tip of the LAA usually points inferiorly and parallel in course with the left anterior descending artery (LAD); however, at times it can be directed posteriorly or into the transverse pericardial sinus.[25]

Anatomic Shapes and Variants
Better spatial and temporal resolution provided by computed tomography and MRI has ultimately led to the development of anatomic morphology classification schemes. There have been 3 arbitrary classification schemes proposed,[29–31] of which Wang's[29] is the most commonly used (and studied in relationship to thromboembolism risk). The first was proposed by Lacomis and colleagues[31] in 2007, in which they described 3 morphologic types based on the orientation and location of the LAA tip (defined as the most distal tissue): type I, where the tip is oriented superiorly and approximately parallel to the main pulmonary artery and left cardiac border; type II, where the tip is oriented

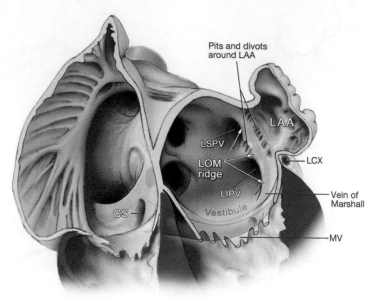

Fig. 2. Endocardial view of the left atrium (LA) and left atrial appendage (LAA), with visualization of the ridge defined by the ligament of Marshall (LOM). The LAA is in close proximity to the left circumflex artery (LCX) as well as the pulmonary veins. CS, coronary sinus; LIPV, left inferior pulmonary vein; LSPV, left superior pulmonary vein; MV, mitral valve. (*Courtesy of* Mayo Foundation for Medical Education and Research, Rochester, MI; with permission.)

inferiorly and approximately parallel to the main pulmonary artery and left cardiac border; and type III, where the tip is oriented superiorly but turning medially and located between the main pulmonary artery and the LA body. Shi and coworkers[30] also proposed a model based on angiography shape in which he proposed 8 morphologic types: tube, claw, spherelike, tadpole, willow leaf, sword, duckbill, and irregular. Wang and associates'[29] morphologic classification is the most commonly used and is established on the bends or angles in the LAA (Fig. 3). It classifies LAA into 2 main morphologic groups based on whether an obvious bend in the proximal/middle part of the dominant lobe was present (chicken wing morphology) or not. Subtypes among the latter category include the windsock (one dominate lobe acts as the primary structure), cactus (dominant central lobe with secondary lobes extending from the central lobe in the superior and inferior directions), and the cauliflower (limited overall length with more complex internal characteristics).

EXTERNAL ANATOMY AND SPATIAL RELATIONSHIPS

The LAA projects from the superior aspect of the LA and is encompassed by the pericardium. In most circumstances, the tip is directed anteriorly and cephalad, where it overlaps with the pulmonary trunk and right ventricular outflow tract. Rarely, the tip may course behind the pulmonary trunk, which consequently precludes the use of epicardial exclusion techniques (see Anatomic Considerations). The LAA shares close spatial relationships (Fig. 4) with critical structures, including multiple blood vessels, nerves, and the mitral valve. A strong understanding of these relationships is, therefore, imperative when considering the appropriateness of LAA exclusion devices and the potential pitfalls that may arise.

Vasculature

The LAA lies close to a number of important vascular structures. The left atrioventricular groove, which houses the LCX and great cardiac

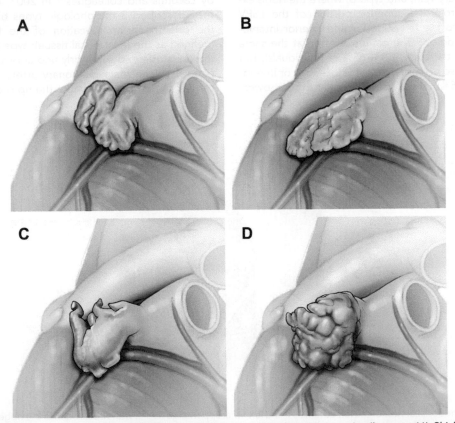

Fig. 3. Morphology classification of the left atrial appendage based on Wang and colleagues. (A) Chicken wing. (B) Windsock. (C) Cactus. (D) Cauliflower. (Courtesy of Mayo Foundation for Medical Education and Research, Rochester, MI; with permission.)

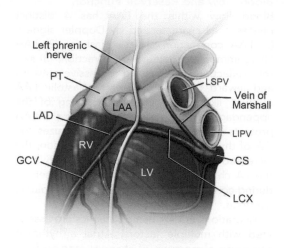

Fig. 4. Epicardial view of the left atrial appendage (LAA) and its spatial relationships with surrounding structures. Note its close proximity to the cardiac vessels and the left phrenic nerve. GCV, great cardiac vein; LAD, left anterior descending artery; LCX, left circumflex artery; LIPV, left inferior pulmonary vein; LSPV, left superior pulmonary vein; LV, left ventricle; PT, pulmonary trunk; RV, right ventricle. (*Courtesy of* Mayo Foundation for Medical Education and Research, Rochester, MI; with permission.)

vein, is positioned inferior to the LAA ostium. The LCX has been shown to run closely (and sometimes in direct contact) with the basal aspect of the LAA orifice.[26] The great cardiac vein, which initially begins as the anterior interventricular vein, enters the left atrioventricular groove as it courses backward and inferiorly around the LA.[32] The LAD has an intimate relationship with the LAA ostium as well, whereby the distance separating the 2 is less than 10 mm in 46% of cases.[14]

Not only are critical arteries in close proximity, but the LSPV lies immediately posterior to the LAA, with part of its anterior wall apposed with the posterior wall of the LAA.[33] The mean distance between the rim of the LAA os and the LPSV was shown to be 11.1 mm (±4.1 mm).[14] Furthermore, the left superior vena cava creates an indentation between the LAA and LSPV during fetal life; this invagination houses the ligament/vein of Marshall (remnant of the left superior vena cava) and defines the left lateral endocardial ridge, which in turn demarcates a physical boundary (superior border) between the LAA and left-sided pulmonary vein ostia.[19,33] Careful consideration of this vasculature should, therefore, be taken into account during exclusion technique planning given their close proximities to the LAA.

Phrenic Nerve

The left phrenic nerve courses along the lateral mediastinum, from the thoracic inlet toward the diaphragm. It is noted to run close to the tip of the LAA or toward the roof of the LAA neck in 59% and 23% of individuals, respectively.[34]

Mitral Valve

The mitral valve is positioned inferior to the LAA ostium, where a vestibule lies interposed between the 2 structures. Given its relatively short separation from the LAA ostium (approximately 11 mm), the mitral valve may be at risk of damage or compression from oversized or malpositioned exclusion devices.[14,19]

INTERNAL ANATOMY

Histology

At the histologic level, the endocardial and epicardial layers of the LAA are interdigitated by a complex mixture of overlapping cardiomyocytes that tend to be oriented in different directions.[19] Three major muscle bundles contribute to its myoarchitecture.[9,35] Subepicardially, Bachmann's bundle bifurcates around the LAA neck and forms a bridging tract between the 2 atria.[36] The septopulmonary bundle fuses with the myocytes from the pulmonary venous muscular sleeves as well as that from the roof and anterior wall of the LAA.[9] Finally, the septoatrial bundle, which forms part of the subendocardium, splits into bands that course close to the LAA opening and into the trabeculations of the pectinate muscles lining its cavity.[9] Between these muscle bundles, the LAA wall thickness can be variable and even paper thin.[37]

Pectinate Muscles and Trabeculations

Unique to the rest of the LA, the endocardial surface of the LAA is lined by a series of fine, rigid pectinate muscles organized in a spiral-like pattern that ultimately creates its characteristic trabeculated appearance.[9,19] In general, trabeculations in the LAA are less pronounced compared with its right-sided counterpart.[38] Larger pectinate muscles are common and can sometimes be mistaken for thrombus on echocardiographic study.[28,39] In addition, extensive trabeculations may be associated with an increased risk of thromboembolism among patients with AF.[40]

Left Atrial Appendage Ostium

The LAA ostium has been recognized to be elliptical and irregular in shape, which contrasts with the rounded features of current LAA exclusion devices. Wang and colleagues[29] categorized LAA ostium shapes into 5 major types using cardiac computed tomography imaging: (1) oval (68.9%); (2) footlike (10.0%); (3) triangular (7.7%); (4) water drop-like (7.7%); and (5) round (5.7%). The average long and short diameters of the orifice measures 17.4 mm and 10.9 mm, respectively[14]; these numbers may vary significantly depending on the imaging modality used and dimensional axes of measure.[28,29,40] The relationship between LAA ostial size and AF is a matter of controversy, as evidenced by the identification of both positive and negative correlations in current literature.[40–42] In addition to LAA orifice dimensions, greater LAA volumes are associated with the presence of AF and thrombi.[43]

PHYSIOLOGIC ROLES

Although the LAA was previously thought to be a vestigial aspect of the heart, several studies have yielded fascinating insights into its physiology. As the use of LAA exclusion devices continues to expand, determining the downstream clinical effects of performing these interventions will be of increasing importance in the near future.

Endocrine Function

Atrial natriuretic peptide (ANP) plays a major role in the regulation of heart rate and volume status.[38] Immunohistochemical studies have demonstrated localization of ANP to the atrial appendages of several mammalian species including humans,[44] suggesting their importance in regulating the storage and release of ANP.[45,46] Indeed, volume status-mediated ANP secretion and consequent renal excretion of salt/fluid were markedly blunted after bilateral atrial appendectomy in canine studies.[44] Recent in-human studies have revealed significant changes in ANP[47] as well as brain natriuretic peptide[48] levels after LAA exclusion. These neurohormonal alterations may be associated with decreases in systolic blood pressure and serum sodium after LAA exclusion[49]; however, further studies will be needed to elucidate this mechanistic link.

Cardiac Progenitor Cell Reservoir

The LAA was found to be a reservoir for cardiac progenitor cells in both murine and human studies.[50–52] These cardiac progenitor cells persist in relatively large numbers during adulthood,[50] suggesting that the LAA may play a significant role in the regeneration of the human heart.

Blood Flow and Reservoir Function

Blood flow within the LAA has 4 distinct phases,[53] as characterized by Doppler signals: (1) LAA contraction at late diastole; (2) LAA filling immediately after LA contraction; (3) systolic reflection waves owing to passive outward and inward flow; and (4) early diastolic LAA outflow, likely from passive emptying of the appendage. This dynamic flow across the LAA protects against hemostasis and minimizes the risk of thrombus formation.[38,53] In addition, the increased compliance of the LAA relative to the LA chamber allows it to act as a reservoir during conditions of LA pressure and/or volume overload.[54]

Alterations in LAA hemodynamics are associated with multiple factors. Atrial arrhythmias can cause a spectrum of changes ranging from relative preservation of LAA contractility to complete paralysis of the appendage.[53,55] Impaired left ventricular filling also significantly affects emptying and filling of the LA as well as the appendage.[53] Additionally, LAA morphology may also have an impact, with the chicken wing shape being associated with higher flow velocities compared with the other types.[56] Decreases in LAA flow and contractility owing to adverse physiologic or morphologic variations increase the propensity for clot development and consequently systemic thromboembolism.[57,58]

CHANGES IN LEFT ATRIAL APPENDAGE ANATOMY WITH ATRIAL FIBRILLATION AND ASSOCIATED INTERVENTIONS

Significant alterations to the normal anatomy of the LAA and its immediate milieu can develop secondary to AF as well as invasive techniques used in its management. A discerning electrophysiologist or interventional cardiologist should, therefore, have a clear understanding of these potential changes and their resulting consequences for LAA exclusion device selection.

Changes with Atrial Fibrillation

The presence of AF is associated with notable changes to LAA anatomy at both the macroscopic and microscopic levels. LAA volume and luminal surface area were higher among patients with AF; by contrast, pectinate muscle surface area and volume were lower.[59] Furthermore, endocardial fibroelastosis[59] and interstitial collagen deposition[60] were more prevalent and severe in the setting of AF. Physiologically, AF is also associated with decreased LAA contractility[61] and flow velocities,[62] as well changes in ANP and inflammatory marker (C-reactive protein) levels.[62,63] Significant individual gene and gene network perturbations have also been noted in the LAA with varying levels of AF severity.[64] In patients with concomitant rheumatic heart disease and AF, inflammatory processes may play a particularly important role, as evidenced by chronic inflammation and fibrotic remodeling noted under gross and microscopic examination.[65] The convergence of these hemodynamic, genetic, and molecular alterations provides conditions amenable to thrombus formation during AF. Additionally, the anatomic remodeling and flow changes associated with AF rhythm can have a major impact on LAA exclusion procedures (see Anatomic Considerations).

Changes After Atrial Fibrillation Catheter Ablation

Catheter ablation has become an increasingly popular choice for the management of symptomatic AF.[66] Although pulmonary vein isolation forms the backbone of AF ablation procedures, there has been recent interest in performing LAA electrical isolation in tandem with standard ablation techniques.[67–69] Not unexpectedly, significant periatrial edema has been noted on cardiac MRI studies after AF ablation; this edema generally abates within 6 months.[70] Improvements in LAA flow/wall velocity and morphology after catheter ablation and restoration of sinus rhythm have also been identified.[70–72] Currently, there is a degree of uncertainty surrounding the efficacy and safety of LAA electrical isolation. Although recurrence rates were lower in LAA electrical isolation plus extensive ablation compared with extensive ablation alone in the BELIEF Trial (Effect of Empirical Left Atrial Appendage Isolation on Long-Term Procedure Outcome in Patients with Persistent or Longstanding Persistent Atrial Fibrillation Undergoing Catheter Ablation), another study found that LAA thrombus formation and cerebrovascular accident rates were higher after LAA electrical isolation.[67,69] Further investigations are therefore needed in assessing these clinical outcomes as well as the mechanisms driving their development.

Changes After Endocardial or Epicardial Device Closure

Although LAA exclusion devices are relatively recent advancements in the management of AF, there is some evidence that these procedures can lead to significant anatomic and functional changes around the region of the LAA. A canine study found that, unlike the Watchman

device, the disc portion of the ACP may interfere with structures adjacent to the LAA ostium, including the LSPV and mitral valve; in addition, although complete neo-endocardial coverage of the Watchman device was noted on histologic study, the ACP remained exposed particularly in the inferior disc edge and end-screw hub.[73] However, there have been no reports of clinically significant device interference with the mitral valve or LSPV in human studies.

With the Lariat approach, strangulation of the epicardial vessels supplying the LAA myocardium promotes transmural necrosis.[74] This process in turn contributes to inflammation and fibrosis at the LAA, ultimately leading to its closure.[75] Incomplete closure is not an uncommon phenomenon; when it occurs, it is associated with a marked reduction in LAA cavity size.[75] The significance of incomplete closure and residual leak after a Lariat procedure is currently incompletely understood, although there have been reports of thrombi developing in the presence of LAA stumps.[76] This factor has led proceduralists to close such leaks with either a repeat Lariat procedure or the Amplatzer Vascular Plug.[77,78]

Postprocedural peridevice leaks (generally defined as a flow >5 mm in width[3,79,80]) differ between the purely endocardial and combined endocardial/epicardial devices. Pillarisetti and colleagues[79] found that postdeployment leaks with the Watchman device tended to be eccentric (ie, around the edges) in nature, in contrast to the centric (gunny-sack–like) leaks observed with the Lariat approach (Fig. 5). Such differences may have a substantial impact on subsequent management, especially in terms of leak closure (as discussed elsewhere in this article) and continuation of anticoagulation therapy.[79] The efficacy and safety of these interventions will need to be investigated further in larger studies.

As procedural techniques continue to mature, there has been increasing interest in the effects of LAA exclusion device placement, either used singly or in combination with catheter ablation, on AF substrate modification. Percutaneous ligation of the LAA may aid in reducing AF burden through a reduction in atrial dispersion[81] and/or removal of LAA substrate and triggers.[82] Initial single[83] and multicenter studies[84] of a combined Watchman device and AF catheter ablation approach demonstrated safety profiles (including postprocedural leaks) and arrhythmia recurrence rates that are comparable with prior trials.[3,85,86] Although promising, further investigations will be needed to assess these techniques' efficacy in mitigating AF among larger groups of patients.

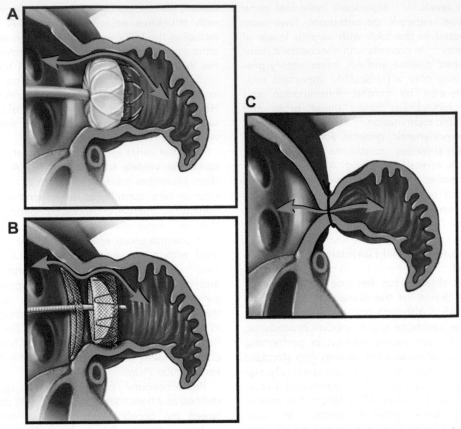

Fig. 5. Peri-device leaks after left atrial appendage closure (*green arrows*). Eccentric flow around the edges of the Watchman (*A*) and Amplatzer Cardiac Plug (*B*), in contrast with the centric leaks ("gunny sack–like") seen with the Lariat device closure (*C*). (*Courtesy of* Mayo Foundation for Medical Education and Research, Rochester, MI; with permission.)

ANATOMIC CONSIDERATIONS FOR CLOSURE

Ostium and Neck

The shape and dimensions of the LAA ostium and neck are essential considerations when it comes to determining the optimal type and size of LAA exclusion device. In terms of the ostium, the majority of LAA ostia tend to be elliptical,[14] which stands in contrast with the rounded profiles of the Watchman device and ACP.[87–93] Peridevice leak owing to ostium–device shape mismatch is, therefore, observed with both implements, although this is somewhat lower with the ACP, possibly owing to its disc-and-plug design as well as the 2 layers of polyester mesh sewn in between.[80,94,95] Interestingly, there has been no significant correlation between the presence of peridevice leaks and adverse clinical outcomes (cardiovascular mortality, stroke, or systemic thromboembolism),[80,94] although further studies will be needed to ensure that these results are borne out. Surrounding structures, including

the mitral valve, LSPV, LAD, and LCX, should be closely examined because these structures can be potentially compromised with device deployment.[9,14] Close attention should be paid to the coronary vasculature in particular. For instance, endocardial device expansion at the ostium can lead to LCX compression.[19] Epicardial tools (for stabilization or looping) positioned near the LAA tip also place the LAD at risk for injury. Additionally, for the ACP, there is a theoretical risk that the disc portion may interfere with the LSPV–LAA ostium or the mitral apparatus, although this has not been observed in clinical studies thus far. Even so, appropriate caution should still be exercised during its sizing and placement.[73]

Sizing for the Watchman device is based on the widest LAA ostial diameter measured, whereas Amplatzer device sizing is determined by the widest diameter measured in the landing zone (10 mm within the orifice for the ACP, 12–15 mm for the Amulet).[96–98] A degree of oversizing is recommended for both devices, with a generally agreed-upon rule of thumb of 10% to 20%.[96,99–101] There are no specific considerations for the Lariat approach in terms of LAA ostial measurements.

In terms of the neck, its long axis diameter can range from 9.5 to 29.9 mm and short axis diameter from 3.1 to 24.0 mm.[102–105] Three different morphologies of the LAA ostium and neck have been described: (1) horn shaped (LAA ostium wider than the neck); (2) parallel tube (ostium and neck similar in dimension); and (3) angel wing (neck with larger dimensions than the LAA ostium).[106] These morphologic

descriptions have significant implications for device/size selection and implantation success because patients with a horn-shaped morphology are believed to have the greatest risk of device dislodgment.

Furthermore, the distance to the first bend has important implications. This is reported to be approximately 14 mm on average; however, in those patients with a chicken wing and cactus morphologic types, they tend to have a shorter overall LAA length and, therefore, the distance to first bend may be shorter. The implication of this is that a small distance long axis-wise can

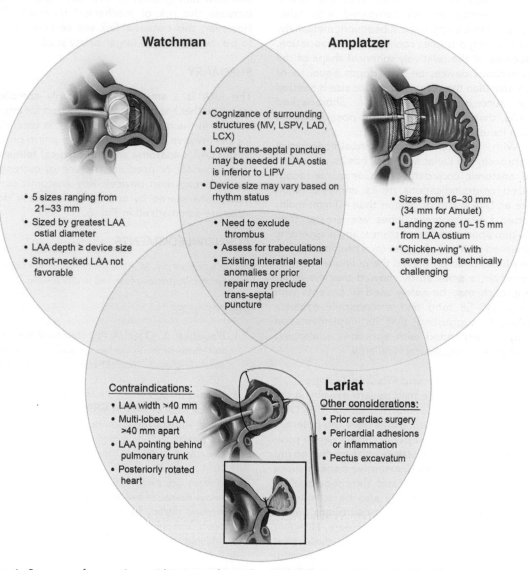

Watchman

- 5 sizes ranging from 21–33 mm
- Sized by greatest LAA ostial diameter
- LAA depth ≥ device size
- Short-necked LAA not favorable

Amplatzer

- Sizes from 16–30 mm (34 mm for Amulet)
- Landing zone 10–15 mm from LAA ostium
- "Chicken-wing" with severe bend technically challenging

- Cognizance of surrounding structures (MV, LSPV, LAD, LCX)
- Lower trans-septal puncture may be needed if LAA ostia is inferior to LIPV
- Device size may vary based on rhythm status

- Need to exclude thrombus
- Assess for trabeculations
- Existing interatrial septal anomalies or prior repair may preclude trans-septal puncture

Lariat

Contraindications:
- LAA width >40 mm
- Multi-lobed LAA >40 mm apart
- LAA pointing behind pulmonary trunk
- Posteriorly rotated heart

Other considerations:
- Prior cardiac surgery
- Pericardial adhesions or inflammation
- Pectus excavatum

Fig. 6. Summary of anatomic considerations relevant for the Watchman, Amplatzer Cardiac Plug, and Lariat devices. LAA, left atrial appendage; LAD, left anterior descending artery; LCX, left circumflex artery; LIPV, left inferior pulmonary vein; LSPV, left superior pulmonary vein; MV, mitral valve. (*Courtesy of* Mayo Foundation for Medical Education and Research, Rochester, MI; with permission.)

increase the risk of perforation by the protruding tip wires.

Morphology, Size, and Position

The morphologic characteristics of the LAA are important to take into account from both prognostic and technical standpoints. Wang's classification schema, as described elsewhere in this article, is probably the most well-studied in these regards[29]; however, variants that depart from such categorizations are not uncommon and should be accounted for by the proceduralist. Lupercio and colleagues[107] and Di Biase and colleagues[108] found that the chicken wing morphology was associated with the lowest thromboembolism risk compared with other morphologic subtypes; a subsequent metaanalysis involving 8 studies confirmed this association. Because of the relatively spherical shape of the Watchman device, an LAA depth equal to or greater than the proposed device size is needed for successful implantation.[87] Short-necked LAAs, therefore, may therefore pose problems with its use.[96,109]

With its combined epicardial/endocardial approach, the Lariat approach has its unique set of anatomic considerations. Commonly recognized contraindications to its implementation are an LAA width of greater than 40 mm; multilobed LAAs whereby lobes are greater than 40 mm apart in different planes; and a superiorly oriented LAA with the apex (or a prominent ancillary lobe) directed behind the pulmonary trunk.[7] However, a small study showed that the Lariat approach may be safely used in patients with large (45–58 mm) and anatomically complex LAAs,[110] suggesting that its implementation may be expanded with appropriate planning and greater procedural familiarity.

Pectinate Muscles and Pits and Troughs

Attention should be paid toward examining the internal anatomic characteristics of the LAA. Prominent pectinate muscles have the potential of interfering with proper occlusion device positioning[96] or being mistaken for thrombus on imaging.[39] As mentioned, extensive trabeculations are associated with greater thromboembolism risk.[40] The LAA ostia may also be surrounded by a variable number of pits/troughs, which tend to be thin walled and, therefore, at higher risk of perforation.[14] In addition, these pits/troughs may not be excluded from the LA circulatory blood flow after the procedure and can remain as persistent niduses for clot formation.[14,19] This remains a potent challenge for current iterations of LAA exclusion devices.

Atrial Fibrillation Severity and Presence at Procedure

Dilatation and fibroelastosis of the LAA occur in the setting of AF, and these changes become more prominent as AF severity increases.[59,111] The increased LAA volumes associated with chronic AF should, therefore, be taken into account when deciding on an appropriate device size. Of note, there were 2 cases of delayed tamponade noted in a recent prospective, single-center study of Watchman and ACP implantation (1 for each device); interestingly, both patients were in sinus rhythm at the time of procedure.[112] The increased LAA contractility and flow during sinus rhythm may theoretically increase the risk of mechanical trauma.[112,113] However, this potential link will certainly need to be investigated in larger safety studies.

SUMMARY

The LAA is a small but remarkably complex structure that has become a key subject for intervention in the management of AF. It is essential for the invasive cardiologist to have a firm grasp of the LAA's anatomy and the physical features that allow for or preclude the use of currently available exclusion devices. Key anatomic considerations shared by and unique to these devices are summarized in **Fig. 6.**

ACKNOWLEDGMENTS

The authors thank M. Alice McKinney for her tireless work on the illustrations featured in this review.

REFERENCES

1. Blackshear JL, Odell JA. Appendage obliteration to reduce stroke in cardiac surgical patients with atrial fibrillation. Ann Thorac Surg 1996;61(2): 755–9.
2. Holmes DR Jr, Kar S, Price MJ, et al. Prospective randomized evaluation of the Watchman Left Atrial Appendage Closure device in patients with atrial fibrillation versus long-term warfarin therapy: the PREVAIL trial. J Am Coll Cardiol 2014;64(1):1–12.
3. Holmes DR, Reddy VY, Turi ZG, et al. Percutaneous closure of the left atrial appendage versus warfarin therapy for prevention of stroke in patients with atrial fibrillation: a randomised non-inferiority trial. Lancet 2009;374(9689):534–42.
4. Tzikas A, Shakir S, Gafoor S, et al. Left atrial appendage occlusion for stroke prevention in atrial fibrillation: multicentre experience with the Amplatzer Cardiac Plug. EuroIntervention 2016; 11(10):1170–9.

5. Freixa X, Chan JL, Tzikas A, et al. The Amplatzer Cardiac Plug 2 for left atrial appendage occlusion: novel features and first-in-man experience. Euro-Intervention 2013;8(9):1094–8.

6. Tzikas A, Gafoor S, Meerkin D, et al. Left atrial appendage occlusion with the AMPLATZER Amulet device: an expert consensus step-by-step approach. EuroIntervention 2016;11(13): 1512–21.

7. Bartus K, Han FT, Bednarek J, et al. Percutaneous left atrial appendage suture ligation using the LARIAT device in patients with atrial fibrillation: initial clinical experience. J Am Coll Cardiol 2013;62(2):108–18.

8. Boersma LV, Schmidt B, Betts TR, et al. Implant success and safety of left atrial appendage closure with the WATCHMAN device: peri-procedural outcomes from the EWOLUTION registry. Eur Heart J 2016;37(31):2465–74.

9. Cabrera JA, Saremi F, Sanchez-Quintana D. Left atrial appendage: anatomy and imaging landmarks pertinent to percutaneous transcatheter occlusion. Heart 2014;100(20):1636–50.

10. Chatterjee S, Herrmann HC, Wilensky RL, et al. Safety and procedural success of left atrial appendage exclusion with the lariat device: a systematic review of published reports and analytic review of the FDA MAUDE database. JAMA Intern Med 2015;175(7):1104–9.

11. Freixa X, Tzikas A, Basmadjian A, et al. The chicken-wing morphology: an anatomical challenge for left atrial appendage occlusion. J Interv Cardiol 2013;26(5):509–14.

12. Lakkireddy D, Afzal MR, Lee RJ, et al. Short and long-term outcomes of percutaneous left atrial appendage suture ligation: results from a US multicenter evaluation. Heart Rhythm 2016;13(5): 1030–6.

13. Matsumoto Y, Morino Y, Kumagai A, et al. Characteristics of anatomy and function of the left atrial appendage and their relationships in patients with cardioembolic stroke: a 3-dimensional trans-esophageal echocardiography study. J Stroke Cerebrovasc Dis 2017;26(3):470–9.

14. Su P, McCarthy KP, Ho SY. Occluding the left atrial appendage: anatomical considerations. Heart 2008;94(9):1166–70.

15. Yuniadi Y, Hanafy DA, Raharjo SB, et al. Amplatzer Cardiac Plug for stroke prevention in patients with atrial fibrillation and bigger left atrial appendix size. Int J Angiol 2016;25(4):241–6.

16. Moorman A, Webb S, Brown NA, et al. Development of the heart: (1) formation of the cardiac chambers and arterial trunks. Heart 2003;89(7): 806–14.

17. Kirby ML. Cardiac development. Oxford (United Kingdom): Oxford University Press; 2007.

18. Kanmanthareddy A, Reddy YM, Vallakati A, et al. Embryology and anatomy of the left atrial appendage: why does thrombus form? Interv Cardiol Clin 2014;3(2):191–202.

19. DeSimone CV, Gaba P, Tri J, et al. A review of the relevant embryology, pathohistology, and anatomy of the left atrial appendage for the invasive cardiac electrophysiologist. J Atr Fibrillation 2015;8(2):81–7.

20. Sherif HM. The developing pulmonary veins and left atrium: implications for ablation strategy for atrial fibrillation. Eur J Cardiothorac Surg 2013; 44(5):792–9.

21. Mirzoyev S, McLeod CJ, Asirvatham SJ. Embryology of the conduction system for the electrophysiologist. Indian Pacing Electrophysiol J 2010; 10(8):329–38.

22. Sedmera D, Pexieder T, Vuillemin M, et al. Developmental patterning of the myocardium. Anat Rec 2000;258(4):319–37.

23. Schmidt B, Ernst S, Ouyang F, et al. External and endoluminal analysis of left atrial anatomy and the pulmonary veins in three-dimensional reconstructions of magnetic resonance angiography: the full insight from inside. J Cardiovasc Electrophysiol 2006;17(9):957–64.

24. Mansour M, Refaat M, Heist EK, et al. Three-dimensional anatomy of the left atrium by magnetic resonance angiography: implications for catheter ablation for atrial fibrillation. J Cardiovasc Electrophysiol 2006;17(7):719–23.

25. Cabrera JA, Ho SY, Climent V, et al. The architecture of the left lateral atrial wall: a particular anatomic region with implications for ablation of atrial fibrillation. Eur Heart J 2008;29(3):356–62.

26. Wongcharoen W, Tsao HM, Wu MH, et al. Morphologic characteristics of the left atrial appendage, roof, and septum: implications for the ablation of atrial fibrillation. J Cardiovasc Electrophysiol 2006;17(9):951–6.

27. Don CW, Cook AC, Reisman M. LAA anatomy. Left atrial appendage closure. New York: Humana Press; 2016. p. 45–57.

28. Veinot JP, Harrity PJ, Gentile F, et al. Anatomy of the normal left atrial appendage: a quantitative study of age-related changes in 500 autopsy hearts: implications for echocardiographic examination. Circulation 1997;96(9):3112–5.

29. Wang Y, Di Biase L, Horton RP, et al. Left atrial appendage studied by computed tomography to help planning for appendage closure device placement. J Cardiovasc Electrophysiol 2010; 21(9):973–82.

30. Shi AW, Chen ML, Yang B, et al. A morphological study of the left atrial appendage in Chinese patients with atrial fibrillation. J Int Med Res 2012; 40(4):1560–7.

31. Lacomis JM, Goitein O, Deible C, et al. Dynamic multidimensional imaging of the human left atrial appendage. Europace 2007;9(12):1134–40.

32. Ho SY, Sanchez-Quintana D, Becker AE. A review of the coronary venous system: a road less travelled. Heart Rhythm 2004;1(1):107–12.

33. Macedo PG, Kapa S, Mears JA, et al. Correlative anatomy for the electrophysiologist: ablation for atrial fibrillation. Part I: pulmonary vein ostia, superior vena cava, vein of Marshall. J Cardiovasc Electrophysiol 2010;21(6):721–30.

34. Sanchez-Quintana D, Ho SY, Climent V, et al. Anatomic evaluation of the left phrenic nerve relevant to epicardial and endocardial catheter ablation: implications for phrenic nerve injury. Heart Rhythm 2009;6(6):764–8.

35. Wang K, Ho SY, Gibson DG, et al. Architecture of atrial musculature in humans. Br Heart J 1995;73(6):559–65.

36. Lemery R, Guiraudon G, Veinot JP. Anatomic description of Bachmann's bundle and its relation to the atrial septum. Am J Cardiol 2003;91(12):1482–5. A1488.

37. Ho SY, Cabrera JA, Sanchez-Quintana D. Left atrial anatomy revisited. Circ Arrhythm Electrophysiol 2012;5(1):220–8.

38. Al-Saady NM, Obel OA, Camm AJ. Left atrial appendage: structure, function, and role in thromboembolism. Heart 1999;82(5):547–54.

39. Baer H, Mereles D, Grunig E, et al. Images in echocardiography. Exaggerated pectinate muscles mimicking multiple left atrial appendage thrombi. Eur J Echocardiogr 2001;2(2):131.

40. Khurram IM, Dewire J, Mager M, et al. Relationship between left atrial appendage morphology and stroke in patients with atrial fibrillation. Heart Rhythm 2013;10(12):1843–9.

41. Beinart R, Heist EK, Newell JB, et al. Left atrial appendage dimensions predict the risk of stroke/TIA in patients with atrial fibrillation. J Cardiovasc Electrophysiol 2011;22(1):10–5.

42. Lee JM, Shim J, Uhm JS, et al. Impact of increased orifice size and decreased flow velocity of left atrial appendage on stroke in nonvalvular atrial fibrillation. Am J Cardiol 2014;113(6):963–9.

43. Ernst G, Stollberger C, Abzieher F, et al. Morphology of the left atrial appendage. Anat Rec 1995;242(4):553–61.

44. Chapeau C, Gutkowska J, Schiller PW, et al. Localization of immunoreactive synthetic atrial natriuretic factor (ANF) in the heart of various animal species. J Histochem Cytochem 1985;33(6):541–50.

45. Hara H, Virmani R, Holmes DR Jr, et al. Is the left atrial appendage more than a simple appendage? Catheter Cardiovasc Interv 2009;74(2):234–42.

46. Syed FF, DeSimone CV, Friedman PA, et al. Left atrial appendage exclusion for atrial fibrillation. Heart Fail Clin 2016;12(2):273–97.

47. Majunke N, Sandri M, Adams V, et al. Atrial and brain natriuretic peptide secretion after percutaneous closure of the left atrial appendage with the Watchman Device. J Invasive Cardiol 2015;27(10):448–52.

48. Cruz-Gonzalez I, Palazuelos Molinero J, Valenzuela M, et al. Brain natriuretic peptide levels variation after left atrial appendage occlusion. Catheter Cardiovasc Interv 2016;87(1):E39–43.

49. Maybrook R, Pillarisetti J, Yarlagadda V, et al. Electrolyte and hemodynamic changes following percutaneous left atrial appendage ligation with the LARIAT device. J Interv Card Electrophysiol 2015;43(3):245–51.

50. Leinonen JV, Emanuelov AK, Platt Y, et al. Left atrial appendages from adult hearts contain a reservoir of diverse cardiac progenitor cells. PLoS One 2013;8(3):e59228.

51. Smits AM, van Vliet P, Metz CH, et al. Human cardiomyocyte progenitor cells differentiate into functional mature cardiomyocytes: an in vitro model for studying human cardiac physiology and pathophysiology. Nat Protoc 2009;4(2):232–43.

52. Winter EM, van Oorschot AA, Hogers B, et al. A new direction for cardiac regeneration therapy: application of synergistically acting epicardium-derived cells and cardiomyocyte progenitor cells. Circ Heart Fail 2009;2(6):643–53.

53. Agmon Y, Khandheria BK, Gentile F, et al. Echocardiographic assessment of the left atrial appendage. J Am Coll Cardiol 1999;34(7):1867–77.

54. Hoit BD, Shao Y, Gabel M. Influence of acutely altered loading conditions on left atrial appendage flow velocities. J Am Coll Cardiol 1994;24(4):1117–23.

55. Garcia-Fernandez MA, Torrecilla EG, San Roman D, et al. Left atrial appendage Doppler flow patterns: implications on thrombus formation. Am Heart J 1992;124(4):955–61.

56. Fukushima K, Fukushima N, Kato K, et al. Correlation between left atrial appendage morphology and flow velocity in patients with paroxysmal atrial fibrillation. Eur Heart J Cardiovasc Imaging 2016;17(1):59–66.

57. Uretsky S, Shah A, Bangalore S, et al. Assessment of left atrial appendage function with transthoracic tissue Doppler echocardiography. Eur J Echocardiogr 2009;10(3):363–71.

58. Goldman ME, Pearce LA, Hart RG, et al. Pathophysiologic correlates of thromboembolism in nonvalvular atrial fibrillation: I. Reduced flow velocity in the left atrial appendage (The Stroke

Prevention in Atrial Fibrillation [SPAF-III] study). J Am Soc Echocardiography 1999;12(12):1080–7.

59. Shirani J, Alaeddini J. Structural remodeling of the left atrial appendage in patients with chronic non-valvular atrial fibrillation: implications for thrombus formation, systemic embolism, and assessment by transesophageal echocardiography. Cardiovasc Pathol 2000;9(2):95–101.

60. Krul SP, Berger WR, Smit NW, et al. Atrial fibrosis and conduction slowing in the left atrial appendage of patients undergoing thoracoscopic surgical pulmonary vein isolation for atrial fibrillation. Circ Arrhythm Electrophysiol 2015;8(2):288–95.

61. Pollick C, Taylor D. Assessment of left atrial appendage function by transesophageal echocardiography. Implications for the development of thrombus. Circulation 1991;84(1):223–31.

62. Yoshida N, Okamoto M, Hirao H, et al. High plasma human atrial natriuretic peptide and reduced transthoracic left atrial appendage wall-motion velocity are noninvasive surrogate markers for assessing thrombogenesis in patients with paroxysmal atrial fibrillation. Echocardiography 2014;31(8):965–71.

63. Cianfrocca C, Loricchio ML, Pelliccia F, et al. C-reactive protein and left atrial appendage velocity are independent determinants of the risk of thrombogenesis in patients with atrial fibrillation. Int J Cardiol 2010;142(1):22–8.

64. Tan N, Chung MK, Smith JD, et al. Weighted gene coexpression network analysis of human left atrial tissue identifies gene modules associated with atrial fibrillation. Circ Cardiovasc Genet 2013;6(4):362–71.

65. Sharma S, Sharma G, Hote M, et al. Light and electron microscopic features of surgically excised left atrial appendage in rheumatic heart disease patients with atrial fibrillation and sinus rhythm. Cardiovasc Pathol 2014;23(6):319–26.

66. January CT, Wann LS, Alpert JS, et al. 2014 AHA/ACC/HRS guideline for the management of patients with atrial fibrillation: executive summary: a report of the American College of Cardiology/American Heart Association Task Force on practice guidelines and the Heart Rhythm Society. Circulation 2014;130(23):2071–104.

67. Di Biase L, Burkhardt JD, Mohanty P, et al. Left atrial appendage isolation in patients with long-standing persistent AF undergoing catheter ablation: BELIEF trial. J Am Coll Cardiol 2016;68(18):1929–40.

68. Hocini M, Shah AJ, Nault I, et al. Localized reentry within the left atrial appendage: arrhythmogenic role in patients undergoing ablation of persistent atrial fibrillation. Heart Rhythm 2011;8(12):1853–61.

69. Rillig A, Tilz RR, Lin T, et al. Unexpectedly high incidence of stroke and left atrial appendage thrombus formation after electrical isolation of the left atrial appendage for the treatment of atrial tachyarrhythmias. Circ Arrhythm Electrophysiol 2016;9(5):e003461.

70. Muellerleile K, Groth M, Steven D, et al. Cardiovascular magnetic resonance demonstrates reversible atrial dysfunction after catheter ablation of persistent atrial fibrillation. J Cardiovasc Electrophysiol 2013;24(7):762–7.

71. Chang SH, Tsao HM, Wu MH, et al. Morphological changes of the left atrial appendage after catheter ablation of atrial fibrillation. J Cardiovasc Electrophysiol 2007;18(1):47–52.

72. Machino-Ohtsuka T, Seo Y, Ishizu T, et al. Significant improvement of left atrial and left atrial appendage function after catheter ablation for persistent atrial fibrillation. Circ J 2013;77(7):1695–704.

73. Kar S, Hou D, Jones R, et al. Impact of Watchman and Amplatzer devices on left atrial appendage adjacent structures and healing response in a canine model. JACC Cardiovasc Interv 2014;7(7):801–9.

74. Turagam M, Atkins D, Earnest M, et al. Anatomical and electrical remodeling with incomplete left atrial appendage ligation: results from the LAALA-AF registry. J Cardiovasc Electrophysiol 2017;28(12):1433–42.

75. Kreidieh B, Rojas F, Schurmann P, et al. Left atrial appendage remodeling after lariat left atrial appendage ligation. Circ Arrhythm Electrophysiol 2015;8(6):1351–8.

76. Price MJ, Gibson DN, Yakubov SJ, et al. Early safety and efficacy of percutaneous left atrial appendage suture ligation: results from the U.S. transcatheter LAA ligation consortium. J Am Coll Cardiol 2014;64(6):565–72.

77. Mosley WJ 2nd, Smith MR, Price MJ. Percutaneous management of late leak after lariat transcatheter ligation of the left atrial appendage in patients with atrial fibrillation at high risk for stroke. Catheter Cardiovasc Interv 2014;83(4):664–9.

78. Pillai AM, Kanmanthareddy A, Earnest M, et al. Initial experience with post Lariat left atrial appendage leak closure with Amplatzer septal occluder device and repeat Lariat application. Heart Rhythm 2014;11(11):1877–83.

79. Pillarisetti J, Reddy YM, Gunda S, et al. Endocardial (Watchman) vs epicardial (Lariat) left atrial appendage exclusion devices: understanding the differences in the location and type of leaks and their clinical implications. Heart Rhythm 2015;12(7):1501–7.

80. Viles-Gonzalez JF, Kar S, Douglas P, et al. The clinical impact of incomplete left atrial appendage

closure with the Watchman Device in patients with atrial fibrillation: a PROTECT AF (percutaneous closure of the left atrial appendage versus warfarin therapy for prevention of stroke in patients with atrial fibrillation) substudy. J Am Coll Cardiol 2012;59(10):923–9.

81. Kawamura M, Scheinman MM, Lee RJ, et al. Left atrial appendage ligation in patients with atrial fibrillation leads to a decrease in atrial dispersion. J Am Heart Assoc 2015;4(5) [pii:e001581].

82. Syed FF, Rangu V, Bruce CJ, et al. Percutaneous ligation of the left atrial appendage results in atrial electrical substrate modification. Transl Res 2015;165(3):365–73.

83. Phillips KP, Walker DT, Humphries JA. Combined catheter ablation for atrial fibrillation and Watchman(R) left atrial appendage occlusion procedures: five-year experience. J Arrhythm 2016;32(2): 119–26.

84. Phillips KP, Pokushalov E, Romanov A, et al. Combining Watchman left atrial appendage closure and catheter ablation for atrial fibrillation: multicentre registry results of feasibility and safety during implant and 30 days follow-up. Europace 2017. https://doi.org/10.1093/europace/eux183.

85. Wilber DJ, Pappone C, Neuzil P, et al. Comparison of antiarrhythmic drug therapy and radiofrequency catheter ablation in patients with paroxysmal atrial fibrillation: a randomized controlled trial. JAMA 2010;303(4):333–40.

86. Parashar A, Tuzcu EM, Kapadia SR. Cardiac plug I and amulet devices: left atrial appendage closure for stroke prophylaxis in atrial fibrillation. J Atr Fibrillation 2015;7(6):1236.

87. Sick PB, Schuler G, Hauptmann KE, et al. Initial worldwide experience with the WATCHMAN left atrial appendage system for stroke prevention in atrial fibrillation. J Am Coll Cardiol 2007;49(13): 1490–5.

88. Masoudi FA, Calkins H, Kavinsky CJ, et al. 2015 ACC/HRS/SCAI left atrial appendage occlusion device societal overview. J Am Coll Cardiol 2015;66(13):1497–513.

89. Reddy VY, Doshi SK, Sievert H, et al. Percutaneous left atrial appendage closure for stroke prophylaxis in patients with atrial fibrillation: 2.3-year follow-up of the PROTECT AF (Watchman left atrial appendage system for embolic protection in patients with atrial fibrillation) trial. Circulation 2013;127(6):720–9.

90. Rodes-Cabau J, Champagne J, Bernier M. Transcatheter closure of the left atrial appendage: initial experience with the Amplatzer Cardiac Plug device. Catheter Cardiovasc Interv 2010; 76(2):186–92.

91. Bass JL. Transcatheter occlusion of the left atrial appendage–experimental testing of a new

Amplatzer device. Catheter Cardiovasc Interv 2010;76(2):181–5.

92. Lam YY, Yip GW, Yu CM, et al. Left atrial appendage closure with AMPLATZER cardiac plug for stroke prevention in atrial fibrillation: initial Asia-Pacific experience. Catheter Cardiovasc Interv 2012;79(5):794–800.

93. Park JW, Bethencourt A, Sievert H, et al. Left atrial appendage closure with Amplatzer cardiac plug in atrial fibrillation: initial European experience. Catheter Cardiovasc Interv 2011;77(5):700–6.

94. Saw J, Tzikas A, Shakir S, et al. Incidence and clinical impact of device-associated thrombus and peri-device leak following left atrial appendage closure with the Amplatzer cardiac plug. JACC Cardiovasc Interv 2017;10(4):391–9.

95. Lopez-Minguez JR, Gonzalez-Fernandez R, Fernandez-Vegas C, et al. Anatomical classification of left atrial appendages in specimens applicable to CT imaging techniques for implantation of Amplatzer cardiac plug. J Cardiovasc Electrophysiol 2014;25(9):976–84.

96. Saw J, Lempereur M. Percutaneous left atrial appendage closure: procedural techniques and outcomes. JACC Cardiovasc Interv 2014;7(11): 1205–20.

97. Bartus K, Bednarek J, Myc J, et al. Feasibility of closed-chest ligation of the left atrial appendage in humans. Heart Rhythm 2011;8(2): 188–93.

98. Lee RJ, Bartus K, Yakubov SJ. Catheter-based left atrial appendage (LAA) ligation for the prevention of embolic events arising from the LAA: initial experience in a canine model. Circ Cardiovasc Interv 2010;3(3):224–9.

99. Alli OO, Holmes DR Jr. Left atrial appendage occlusion for stroke prevention. Curr Probl Cardiol 2015;40(10):429–76.

100. Shah SJ, Bardo DM, Sugeng L, et al. Real-time three-dimensional transesophageal echocardiography of the left atrial appendage: initial experience in the clinical setting. J Am Soc Echocardiography 2008; 21(12):1362–8.

101. Sommer M, Roehrich A, Boenner F, et al. Value of 3D TEE for LAA morphology. JACC Cardiovasc Imaging 2015;8(9):1107–10.

102. Heist EK, Refaat M, Danik SB, et al. Analysis of the left atrial appendage by magnetic resonance angiography in patients with atrial fibrillation. Heart Rhythm 2006;3(11):1313–8.

103. Blendea D, Heist EK, Danik SB, et al. Analysis of the left atrial appendage morphology by intracardiac echocardiography in patients with atrial fibrillation. J Interv Card Electrophysiol 2011;31(3): 191–6.

104. Otton JM, Spina R, Sulas R, et al. Left atrial appendage closure guided by personalized

3D-printed cardiac reconstruction. JACC Cardiovasc Interv 2015;8(7):1004–6.

105. Pellegrino PL, Fassini G, Di Biase M, et al. Left atrial appendage closure guided by 3D printed cardiac reconstruction: emerging directions and future trends. J Cardiovasc Electrophysiol 2016; 27(6):768–71.

106. Yu CM, Khattab AA, Bertog SC, et al. Mechanical antithrombotic intervention by LAA occlusion in atrial fibrillation. Nat Rev Cardiol 2013;10(12): 707–22.

107. Lupercio F, Carlos Ruiz J, Briceno DF, et al. Left atrial appendage morphology assessment for risk stratification of embolic stroke in patients with atrial fibrillation: a meta-analysis. Heart Rhythm 2016; 13(7):1402–9.

108. Di Biase L, Santangeli P, Anselmino M, et al. Does the left atrial appendage morphology correlate with the risk of stroke in patients with atrial fibrillation? Results from a multicenter study. J Am Coll Cardiol 2012;60(6):531–8.

109. Ismail TF, Panikker S, Markides V, et al. CT imaging for left atrial appendage closure: a review and pictorial essay. J Cardiovasc Comput Tomogr 2015;9(2):89–102.

110. Patel MB, Rasekh A, Shuraih M, et al. Safety and effectiveness of compassionate use of LARIAT(R) device for epicardial ligation of anatomically complex left atrial appendages. J Interv Card Electrophysiol 2015;42(1):11–9.

111. Park HC, Shin J, Ban JE, et al. Left atrial appendage: morphology and function in patients with paroxysmal and persistent atrial fibrillation. Int J Cardiovasc Imaging 2013;29(4):935–44.

112. Chun KR, Bordignon S, Urban V, et al. Left atrial appendage closure followed by 6 weeks of antithrombotic therapy: a prospective single-center experience. Heart Rhythm 2013;10(12): 1792–9.

113. Perrotta L, Bordignon S, Dugo D, et al. Complications from left atrial appendage exclusion devices. J Atr Fibrillation 2014;7(1):1034.

The WATCHMAN Left Atrial Appendage Closure Device
Technical Considerations and Procedural Approach

Matthew J. Price, MD

KEYWORDS

- Left atrial appendage • Stroke • Atrial fibrillation • WATCHMAN

KEY POINTS

- Procedural safety is paramount, as LAA closure for stroke prevention is a prophylactic procedure that is often performed in elderly patients with multiple co-morbidities in whom procedural complications may not be well-tolerated.
- A complication rate <2% can be achieved with a fastidious approach that incorporates the lessons learned from early experience.
- The appropriate device size should be selected by synthesizing the maximal ostial diameters by TEE and cardiac CT imaging (if performed), and cineangiography when the access sheath is positioned deep within the LAA.
- Comprehensive TEE evaluation after implantation and before device release can identify residual leaks, large posterior shoulders, and uncovered lobes, all of which are unacceptable and may place the patient at risk for device embolism, large peri-device flow at follow-up that requires long-term OAC, and/or thromboembolic events if OAC is discontinued.

INTRODUCTION

Randomized clinical trials have demonstrated that left atrial appendage (LAA) closure with the WATCHMAN device (Boston Scientific, Inc, Marlborough, MA, USA) provides stroke prevention in nonvalvular atrial fibrillation (AF), similar to the vitamin K-antagonist warfarin, while significantly reducing mortality and major bleeding.[1,2] Technical and procedural considerations are paramount for the therapeutic success of LAA closure. First, optimal LAA sealing is required because the LAA is the predominant source of thromboembolism in AF, and the goal of LAA closure is to remove this source from the circulation.[3] This may not be straightforward in all cases given the combination of LAA anatomic variability[4] and the WATCHMAN

mechanism of action. The WATCHMAN device occludes the LAA from within and, therefore, successful closure depends critically on the interaction between the device and LAA anatomy, including but not limited to LAA ostial width; lobe depth; the presence, location, size, and rigidity of septae dividing lobes; the distribution of trabeculations; and anterior or posterior orientation of the main LAA body. In addition, maximizing procedural safety is critical because the rate of procedural complications influences clinical decision-making and patient selection for transcatheter LAA closure or for chronic oral anticoagulation (OAC). Three sources of risk must be incorporated: the risk of procedural complications with LAA closure, the individual's thromboembolic risk without OAC treatment (derived from well-established

---

Division of Cardiovascular Diseases, Scripps Clinic, 9898 Genesee Avenue, AMP-200, La Jolla, CA 92037, USA
E-mail address: price.matthew@scrippshealth.org

Intervent Cardiol Clin 7 (2018) 201–212
https://doi.org/10.1016/j.iccl.2017.12.010
2211-7458/18/© 2017 Elsevier Inc. All rights reserved.

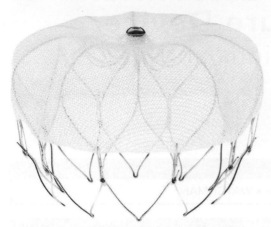

Fig. 1. The WATCHMAN LAA closure device. The device comprises a self-expanding nitinol frame with a polyethylene terephthalate fabric cap. Distal fixation anchors secure the device within the LAA trabeculae. (Image provided *courtesy of* Boston Scientific. ©2018 Boston Scientific Corporation or its affiliates. All rights reserved.)

risk-stratification schemes, such as the CHA$_2$DS$_2$-VASc score[5]), and the individual's long-term bleeding risk with OAC treatment. Improvements in procedural technique and operator training have resulted in a marked reduction in adverse procedural events[6,7] and procedural success rates of greater than 98%,[8] which may increase the absolute clinical benefit for patients over the long-term. This article outlines the key aspects of patient workup and procedural techniques that will result in the best possible outcomes.

WATCHMAN DEVICE AND DELIVERY SHEATH CHARACTERISTICS

Device

The WATCHMAN is made of a self-expanding nitinol frame with a polyethylene terephthalate fabric 160 μm mesh cap that faces the left atrial chamber (Fig. 1). The fabric cap covers about one-half of the proximal portion of the device. Available sizes are 21 mm, 24 mm, 27 mm, 30 mm, and 33 mm; the device size corresponds to the width of the unconstrained device at its proximal shoulders. Most of the radial strength of the device is located at these shoulders. The length of the device is approximately equal to its width. Fixation anchors, located just distal to the distal end of the polyester fabric cap, secure the device within the LAA trabeculae. The device attaches to a delivery cable at a central, threaded insert.

Delivery Sheath

The WATCHMAN device is delivered through a 14F access sheath. This access sheath has 4 radiopaque marker bands (Fig. 2): the distal-most marker band defines the distal end of the sheath and the proximal 3 marker bands act as landmarks for estimating the proximal landing site of the device after the sheath has been introduced into the LAA. The sheath comes in 3 shapes: double, single, and anterior curve (Fig. 3). The double-curve sheath is sufficient to provide depth and coaxial orientation within the LAA in most cases. The single-curve sheath may be advantageous if there is a single (or

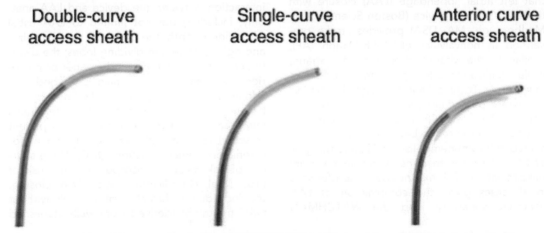

| Double-curve access sheath | Single-curve access sheath | Anterior curve access sheath |

Fig. 2. The WATCHMAN access sheath. The 14F WATCHMAN access sheath is available in 3 shapes: double-curve (*left*), single-curve (*middle*), and anterior curve (*right*). The double-curve sheath is sufficient to provide depth and coaxial orientation within the LAA in most cases. The single-curve sheath may be advantageous when there is a single or dominant posterior lobe. The anterior curve sheath is helpful to achieve a coaxial position when the LAA has a markedly anterior orientation. (Image provided *courtesy of* Boston Scientific. ©2018 Boston Scientific Corporation or its affiliates. All rights reserved.)

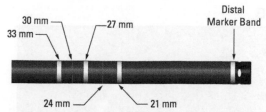

Fig. 3. WATCHMAN access sheath marker bands. The more distal marker signifies the estimated landing site of a 21-mm device, the middle marker a 27-mm device, and the proximal marker a 33-mm device. For example, if the goal is to implant a 27-mm device (based on TEE measurements), the sheath must be advanced deeply enough into the LAA so that the middle marker is at or just distal to the LAA ostium. (Image provided *courtesy of* Boston Scientific. ©2018 Boston Scientific Corporation or its affiliates. All rights reserved.)

dominant) posterior lobe. The anterior curve sheath is helpful to achieve a coaxial position if the LAA has a markedly anterior orientation.

PREPROCEDURAL EVALUATION

Anatomic Evaluation for Feasibility

Assessment of LAA size and shape is required to determine the feasibility of WATCHMAN implantation because the LAA ostial width must be adequate to provide appropriate device compression (8% to 20%). Simultaneously, there must be sufficient depth to accommodate the device, which is dictated by that width (the device length is roughly the same as its diameter). Preprocedural transesophageal echocardiography (TEE) was used to assess LAA anatomy in randomized clinical trials that demonstrated device safety and efficacy compared with warfarin.[1,2,6,9] Key features that should be identified on preprocedural TEE are listed in **Box 1**.

The LAA ostium is formed superiorly by the limbus of left upper pulmonary vein (LUPV) and inferiorly by the area adjacent to the mitral valve annulus and above the left atrioventricular groove, which contains the left circumflex artery.[10] The LAA ostial diameter is defined as the distance from a point just distal to the left circumflex artery to approximately 1 to 2 cm from the tip of the LUPV limbus. Alternatively, the LAA ostium can be measured by drawing a line from the mitral valve annulus across to the LUPV, perpendicular to the planned axis of the delivery sheath. The LAA depth is defined as the distance from the midpoint of the line that defines the ostium to the deepest point within the LAA, preferably at the apex of the

> **Box 1**
> **Features that should be identified on baseline imaging before WATCHMAN device implantation**
>
> - LAA thrombus (if present, LAA closure should be deferred until addressed)
> - Maximum diameter of the LAA ostium
> - Maximum LAA depth
> - LAA shape (in particular, chicken wing)
> - Presence of thickened, rigid septae that might interfere with full device expansion
> - Presence and magnitude of pericardial effusion, if any, to serve as baseline reference device implantation
> - Abnormalities of the interatrial septum that might interfere with transseptal puncture (eg, large patent foramen ovale, significant lipomatous hypertrophy)
> - Presence of conditions that require long-term OAC (eg, mobile aortic atheroma or left ventricular thrombus, mitral stenosis)

anterior-most lobe. The LAA is imaged and these ostial and depth measurements taken in a systematic fashion from the midesophageal view at 0°, 45°, 90°, and 135° (**Fig. 4**). The patient may not be a candidate for closure if the maximal LAA depth on TEE is not sufficient for the smallest acceptable device based on the maximal LAA ostial diameter (ie, the LAA is shallow and wide) or if the ostium is too wide or narrow for the largest or smallest device (in general, >30 mm or <17 mm, respectively).

Rather than using 2-dimensional (D) TEE to determine the LAA ostial diameters (which dictates device size selection), investigators have proposed using multiplanar reconstruction (MPR) of the LAA ostium by TEE or cardiac computed tomography (CT), as well as 3-D–derived LAA ostial area and perimeter to guide device size selection.[11,12] The LAA ostial diameter by MPR CT is, on average, approximately 2 to 3 mm larger than by 2-D TEE.[12,13] Early studies have shown that these approaches may improve the efficiency of device selection (eg, reducing the number of devices used per case). However, more study is required to robustly determine whether these techniques improve procedure success and patient outcomes compared with the standard TEE approach proscribed in the randomized clinical trials that led to WATCHMAN approval. More aggressive oversizing based on 2-D TEE measurements, particularly when the measurement lands at the

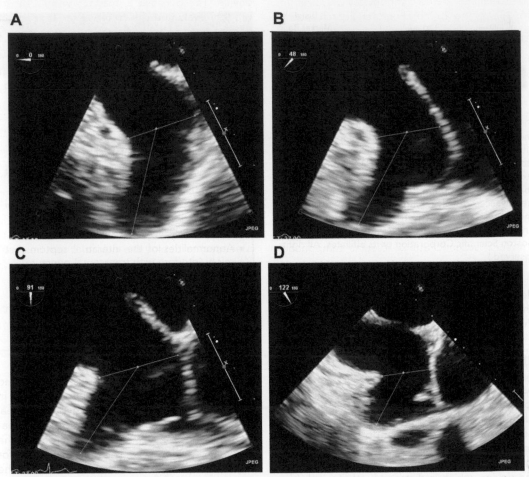

Fig. 4. Preprocedural TEE assessment of the LAA for WATCHMAN implantation. TEE is performed before the procedure to exclude the presence of LAA thrombus and to confirm that LAA anatomy is feasible for occlusion. The diameter and depth of the LAA is measured at 0° (A), 45° (B), 90° (C), and 135° (D). The diameter of the LAA is defined as the distance from a point just distal to the left circumflex artery to roughly 1 to 2 cm from the tip of the LUPV limbus. An initial device size is selected to be at least 10% to 20% greater than the maximal width, provided there is sufficient depth. The decision on device size may be adjusted after fluoroscopic landmarks are obtained and while the access sheath is advanced deep within the LAA. In this case, the LAA has a modest anterior chicken-wing morphology, which may increase procedural complexity but does not preclude procedural success. Alternative approaches to define LAA ostial diameters and optimal WATCHMAN device size include CT imaging and 3-D TEE multiplanar reconstruction, although the advantages of these methods with respect to safety and efficacy have not been robustly evaluated. (*Adapted from* Price MJ. Left atrial appendage occlusion with the WATCHMAN™ for stroke prevention in atrial fibrillation. Rev Cardiovasc Med 2014;15:145; with permission.)

border zone between 2 sizes, may be sufficient to compensate for the modest undersizing compared with cardiac CT. In 1 study, routine CT identified subjects who would have been excluded from WATCHMAN implantation by TEE.[12] Therefore, preprocedural CT imaging should be strongly considered in cases in which the LAA is poorly visualized by TEE. A practical approach is to perform preprocedural CT to confirm anatomic eligibility, and to use multimodality imaging (preprocedural CT, intraprocedural TEE, and fluoroscopy) to select the appropriate sized device during the procedure itself (see later discussion).

PROCEDURAL STEPS

The procedural steps can be summarized as baseline TEE imaging, venous access, transseptal puncture (TSP), advancement of the access sheath into the LAA, device size selection and implantation, evaluation of implantation result, and release and withdrawal of the equipment.

Preprocedural Anticoagulation

In the WATCHMAN Left Atrial Appendage System for Embolic Protection in Patients with Atrial Fibrillation (PROTECT-AF) and the Prospective Randomized Evaluation of the WATCHMAN Left Atrial Appendage Closure Device In Patients with Atrial Fibrillation vs Long-Term Warfarin Therapy (PREVAIL) clinical trials, the protocol did not specify the management of the immediate preprocedural anticoagulation regimen.[6,9] Many operators discontinue warfarin and non-vitamin K OACs (NOACs) before LAA closure to minimize the sequelae of pericardial effusion if it were to occur. A periprocedural pericardial effusion might be particularly difficult to manage in a patient treated with oral direct factor X inhibitors, which currently have no reversal agent. However, a strategy of routine OAC or NOAC discontinuation before LAA closure may increase the risk of LAA thrombus at the time of the procedure. In a retrospective multicenter study, uninterrupted or single-held dose NOAC was associated with a similar rate of periprocedural complications, including bleeding events, as uninterrupted warfarin therapy (2.8% vs 2.4%, respectively).[14] The decision to hold warfarin or NOAC before the procedure should depend on several factors, including operator comfort and patient thromboembolic risk.

Preprocedural Imaging

Before venous access, TEE imaging should be performed to exclude the presence of LAA thrombus, which is a contraindication for LAA closure. The anatomic feasibility for closure should also be assessed if this was not done by TEE before the day of the procedure. If a baseline TEE was performed, the anatomy and size measurements should be confirmed because the echocardiographic visualization of the LAA may change in the supine position under general anesthesia.

Venous Access

Right femoral venous access is established with a standard introducer sheath, usually 8F. The vein can be preclosed with a Perclose device (Abbott Vascular, Santa Clara, CA, USA); alternatively, a figure-of-8 stitch at the end of the procedure can be used, eliminating the need and associated cost of a closure device. At the authors' site, the 8F sheath is then upsized to a 16F sheath, through which TSP is performed, and then the 14F access sheath is introduced. The 16F sheath eliminates resistance at the groin during fine manipulation of the access sheath in the LAA and is particularly helpful when the

pelvic veins are highly tortuous, the subcutaneous tissue scarred due to prior procedures, or when there is significant obesity. Moreover, the 16F sheath can maintain venous access and hemostasis if atrial balloon septostomy is required to pass the large access sheath across the interatrial septum. This large sheath can also serve as large bore access in case of hemodynamic compromise and/or tamponade, and blood can be drawn through it to measure activated clotting time (ACT) during the procedure. Alternatively, a 5F sheath can be placed in the contralateral femoral vein or large bore intravenous access obtained for secondary venous access. In general, the authors prefer to avoid venous access in the neck to improve patient comfort postprocedure and to minimize anesthesia setup time.

Anticoagulation

Unfractionated heparin (UFH) is used to achieve therapeutic anticoagulation during the procedure, with a goal ACT of at least 250 to 300 seconds. Some operators give full-dose UFH as soon as venous access is obtained; some wait until successful intravenous TSP is performed; and others administer a half-dose of UFH after placement of the venous sheath and before TSP, and then administer the remainder after entry into the left atrium. Although waiting until after successful TSP may theoretically reduce the risk of uncontrolled pericardial effusion, this approach might increase the risk of thrombus formation on wires and equipment within the left atrium. An ACT should be obtained frequently to ensure appropriate anticoagulation is maintained for the duration of the procedure.

Transseptal Puncture

TSP should be performed under TEE guidance, preferably with multiplane imaging for simultaneous visualization of the long and short axes of the interatrial septum (Fig. 5). For LAA closure, the TSP site should be located inferiorly and posteriorly because this orients the access sheath coaxially with the LAA (Fig. 6). On occasion, a more optimal TSP may be located more in the midseptum rather than inferiorly. The need for a less inferior TSP can be identified by examining the TEE 90° view of the LAA. When the body of the LAA is directed steeply downward, parallel to the body of the left ventricle, this signifies a more posteriorly directed appendage and, therefore, deep intubation of the LAA will be challenging with a very inferior puncture.

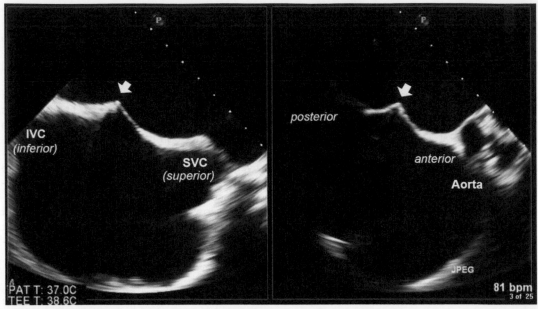

Fig. 5. TEE guidance of TSP. The exact location of the TSP along the interatrial septum can be visualized by simultaneous imaging of the bicaval (*left*) and aortic (*right*) short-axis planes using a 3-D probe. For LAA closure, a posterior-inferior puncture is advantageous because it allows for a coaxial approach for equipment to be introduced into the LAA. In this particular case, the transseptal dilator is tenting the midportion of the interatrial septum. Arrows: tenting of interatrial septum by the transseptal sheath dilator. IVC, inferior vena cava; SVC, superior vena cava. (*Adapted from* Price MJ, Smith MR, Rubenson DS, et al. Catheter-based left atrial appendage closure. In: Picard MH, Passeri JJ, Dal-Biancoet JP, editors. Intraprocedural imaging of cardiovascular interventions. 1st edition. Switzerland: Springer; 2016. p. 109; with permission.)

After TSP is successful, the transseptal sheath is exchanged for the 14F access sheath. This can be done over a 0.25 in Inouye-type wire such as the ProTrack Pigtail (Baylis Medical, Montreal, Canada) or an 0.35 in extra-stiff Amplatz wire placed within the LUPV. Introduction of the extra-stiff wire into the LAA should be fastidiously avoided because this can result in cardiac perforation, particularly during sheath exchanges. The ProTrack wire has a flexible, spiral tip with a supportive body, which facilitates catheter exchanges by maintaining left atrial access and reducing the risk of perforation; this is the preferred wire for all left atrial sheath exchanges at the authors' institution.

Delivery Sheath Selection

The WATCHMAN access sheath is available in 3 shapes: double, single, and anterior curve. The double-curve sheath is sufficient to provide depth and coaxial orientation within the LAA in most cases. The single-curve sheath is advantageous when there is a single (or dominant) posterior lobe. The anterior curve sheath is helpful to achieve a coaxial position when the LAA has a markedly anterior orientation. The anterior curve sheath should be used cautiously: if it is used to achieve greater depth within a so-called chicken wing that is anteriorly directed, the introduction of the WATCHMAN device into the distal end of the sheath will straighten the curve and risk laceration of the outer wall of the LAA.

Advancement of Delivery Sheath into the Left Atrial Appendage

The access sheath and dilator are advanced over the stiff wire anchored within the LUPV (or the Inouye-type wire within the left atrium). Rotation of the access sheath so that its side-port points in approximately the 3 o'clock direction (in which 12 o'clock is the direction toward the ceiling) will generally provide a coaxial orientation to more easily deliver the sheath and dilator across the septum. Simultaneous TEE imaging of the basal short axis of the interatrial septum can monitor the sheath as it crosses the septum: persistent tenting of the interatrial septum will occur if the sheath or dilator cannot fully cross because of a recalcitrant, thick, or floppy septum. In this case, the sheath and dilator should be

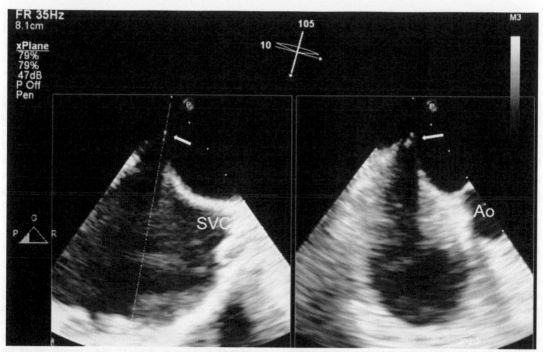

Fig. 6. Optimal transseptal location for WATCHMAN LAA occlusion. The tenting of the septum by the transseptal needle is inferior, on the opposite end of the interatrial septum from the SVC (*left*) and posterior (opposite) to the aortic valve (*right*). This directs the device delivery sheath toward the LAA in a coaxial fashion because the appendage is located in the anterior and superior portion of the left atrium. Arrows: tenting of interatrial septum by transseptal needle. Ao, aorta. (*Adapted from* Price MJ, Smith MR, Rubenson DS, et al. Catheter-based left atrial appendage closure. In: Picard MH, Passeri JJ, Dal-Biancoet JP, editors. Intraprocedural imaging of cardiovascular interventions. 1st edition. Switzerland: Springer; 2016. p. 109; with permission.)

withdrawn over the wire and a balloon septostomy performed with at least a 5.0 by 40-mm balloon to dilate the septum sufficiently for sheath crossing.

After the wire and dilator are removed, the access sheath should be carefully flushed with saline. The operator must be meticulous in preventing the introduction of air within the sheath and subsequently the left atrium because this is the primary cause of procedure-related stroke. Air embolism was in large part responsible for procedure-related ischemic strokes in the early part of the PROTECT-AF trial, which in part contributed to the numerically higher rates of ischemic stroke in the device arm of that trial.[7,9] A 6F straight pigtail catheter is then introduced into the sheath, advanced into the left atrium, and connected to the manifold for contrast injections. Left atrial pressure should be measured at this juncture (if it was not measured at the time of TSP). A mean left atrial pressure greater than or equal to 10 mm Hg is recommended before device deployment so that LAA size is not underestimated. Boluses of normal saline should be administered until

the goal left atrial pressure is achieved. The operator then intubates the LAA deeply with the pigtail catheter; this is often facilitated by gentle counterclockwise (anterior) rotation of the sheath and pigtail catheter under TEE guidance; in the right anterior oblique (RAO)-caudal projection, the pigtail should be directed up and to the right. LAA angiography is then performed through the pigtail catheter in this RAO-caudal projection, which is the fluoroscopic equivalent of the TEE 135° view; that is, it lays out the LAA in short axis so that the entire breadth of the ostium is visualized. The pigtail catheter should be advanced deeply into the lobe that will provide the greatest depth while coaxially deploying the occluder; this is generally, but not always, the most anterior lobe. The operator then advances the access sheath carefully over the pigtail until adequate depth is obtained for the planned device size. The pigtail catheter acts as a support rail and helps prevent the tip of the delivery sheath from contacting the LAA wall despite deep engagement. Gentle counterclockwise (anterior) rotation of the sheath may facilitate this maneuver by directing the sheath anteriorly, unless there is a single or dominant posterior lobe, in which case clockwise rotation of the sheath may be required to gain adequate depth to implant a device large enough to cover the LAA ostium. Advancing the access sheath over a stiff wire placed in the LAA is not recommended given the risk of LAA perforation, pericardial effusion, and tamponade. Systematic use of a pigtail catheter rail has been an important factor in reducing the periprocedural complication rate of WATCHMAN LAA closure.[7,15]

In some instances, the sheath cannot be advanced sufficiently deep into the LAA because the approach angle is not sufficiently coaxial with the LAA body or the direction of optimal deployment. A single-curve access sheath may be preferred when there is a dominant posterior lobe. In addition, a relatively more superior TSP location may provide a more coaxial approach into the LAA in this situation. When the sheath cannot be directed sufficiently anteriorly, an anterior curve access sheath or a more inferior TSP may provide a better sheath position (Fig. 7). Rarely, when the septum is rigid and/or thick, aggressive rotation may lead to kinking of the access sheath at the site of transseptal crossing. In this situation, the sheath should be removed over a wire, a balloon septostomy performed (see previous discussion), and a new access sheath advanced into the LAA for device deployment.

Final Device Size Selection

The appropriate device size should be selected by synthesizing the maximal ostial diameters by TEE and cardiac CT imaging (if performed), and cineangiography when the access sheath is positioned deep within the LAA. The TEE images should be used to identify the minimally acceptable device size that is approximately 10% to 20% greater than the maximal width of the LAA ostium (Table 1). For example, if the maximal LAA ostial diameter on TEE is 20 mm, the minimal acceptable device size is 24 mm. However, the operator should also incorporate the achievable access sheath depth to optimize size selection. The 3 radiopaque markers act as landmarks to estimate the proximal landing site of the WATCHMAN device if it is to be deployed at the current location of the access sheath (see Fig. 3). The most distal of the 3 markers signifies the estimated landing site of a 21-mm device, the middle marker a 27-mm device, and the proximal marker a 33-mm device. For example, if the goal is to implant a 27-mm device, the sheath must be advanced deeply enough into the LAA so that the middle marker is at or just distal to the LAA ostium (determined by angiography). Many operators choose the largest device that can be implanted based on sheath depth as long as it not so big that it is grossly oversized (eg, ≥30%–35% of the maximal ostial diameter by TEE) or smaller than the minimally acceptable device size previously described (Fig. 8). Severe oversizing of the device can

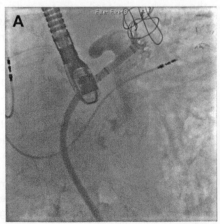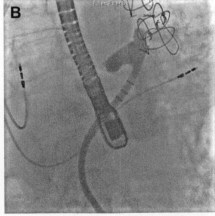

Fig. 7. Influence of TSP location on sheath delivery into the LAA. (*A*) The double-curve access sheath cannot be positioned deep within the LAA because it is not coaxial with the LAA ostium, even after substantial counterclockwise rotation. (*B*) Coaxial orientation with the LAA is obtained by performing another TSP more inferiorly than the first, and switching to an anterior curve access sheath. A WATCHMAN 24-mm device was successfully implanted. (*Adapted from* Price MJ. Left atrial appendage therapies. In: Kern M, Lim M, Sorajja P, editors. The interventional cardiac catheterization handbook. 4th edition. Philadelphia: Elsevier; 2018. p. 482; with permission.)

Table 1 Compression table for WATCHMAN device sizing	
Device Size (mm)	**Deployed Diameter (mm)**
21	16.8–19.3
24	19.2–22.1
27	21.6–24.8
30	24.0–27.6
33	26.4–30.4

result in too much compression, which may lead to (1) instability and embolism because the distal fixation anchors may not fully open, and (2) peridevice leak due to dimpling of the circumference of the polyester fabric caps such that it will be unopposed to the LAA wall.

Device Deployment

An optimal access sheath position should be obtained before introducing the WATCHMAN device. This optimal position is defined by (1) adequate depth to implant the appropriately sized device (see previous discussion) and (2) an appropriate coaxial orientation with the LAA ostium, achieved by rotation of the access sheath either anteriorly (in a counterclockwise fashion) or posteriorly (in a clockwise fashion). Although the optimal orientation of the sheath will most commonly be anterior, clockwise rotation of the sheath may be required to achieve

sufficient depth when there is a single or dominant posterior lobe. In this case, care must be taken to avoid leaving the device with a large posterior shoulder (protrusion into the left atrium) due to the device's horizontal orientation.

After optimal sheath position is obtained, the manifold is connected to the flush port of the delivery system, ventilation is held, and the pigtail catheter removed. The delivery system, which contains the preloaded device, is flushed to remove any air, introduced into the access sheath, and advanced until the radio-opaque marker of the distal end of the delivery system is aligned with the distal marker of the access sheath. Filling the access sheath with contrast after introducing the delivery system can help visualize the relationship between the distal end of the sheath and the back wall of the LAA; however, care must be taken not to introduce air into the system during this maneuver. The operator must also maintain any torque on the access sheath while advancing the device so as to maintain optimal access sheath position. After the markers are aligned, the operator stabilizes the proximal end of the delivery system and retracts the access sheath so that it snaps into the delivery system, creating a single assembly. The operator loosens the valve on the delivery system, holds the deployment knob stable, and retracts the access sheath delivery system assembly to unsheathe and deploy the self-expanding device.

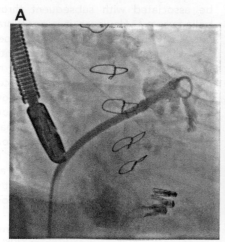 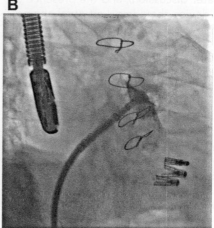

Fig. 8. Device sizing. In this patient, the 2-D TEE–derived maximal LAA ostial diameter and maximal LAA depth was 25 mm and 34 mm, respectively. Therefore, the minimally acceptable device size would be 30 mm (approximately 20% oversized). (A) The sheath was easily advanced deep within the LAA so that the most proximal marker of the access sheath (signifying the landing site of a 33-mm device) was aligned with the angiographic LAA ostium. (B) A WATCHMAN 33-mm device was selected and implanted, resulting in excellent device position (no posterior shoulder) and optimal compression by TEE and fluoroscopy.

It is imperative that the distal end of the device (the feet) remain fixed in position and not move forward because this could cause tearing of the friable LAA wall, nor should the feet fall back because this will result in a proximal device deployment. Proximal displacement of the feet can be avoided by gentle counterpressure on the deployment knob while the access sheath delivery system assembly is retracted. This counterpressure is particularly important when the shoulders of the device are released because this represents the point of greatest radial expansion of the device and is the most common moment for proximal displacement to occur. It can be helpful to perform device implantation under cineangiography or to store the fluoroscopic run directly after implantation so that, if the implantation is unsuccessful, the mechanisms of failure can be identified (eg, suboptimal initial position, proximal displacement of the access sheath or feet during deployment, inability of the distal anchors to engage in the LAA wall due to a large diameter lobe).

If the device position after deployment appears acceptable, a tug-test is performed. The tug-test is considered adequate if resistance is felt when pulling back the deployment knob and if the device does not move within the LAA. Additionally, the LAA and the WATCHMAN device should move in unison. Final TEE and angiography is then performed to assess device position. Comprehensive TEE evaluation should assess for peridevice leak, lack of coverage of any lobes, device compression (see later discussion), and the presence of significant device shoulders. Left atrial angiography in RAO-caudal projection is optimal to delineate the relationship between the device and the LAA ostium, including whether all lobes are covered. If required, the anterior posterior (AP)-caudal projection can be used to further interrogate the relationship between the inferior-posterior aspect of the device and the LAA ostium, whereas the AP-cranial projection can be used to interrogate the superior-anterior aspect of the device. Uncovered trabeculations along the limbus of the LUPV that are undetectable by TEE are commonly identified on left atrial angiography after deployment, and may not be covered by the device because they sit outside the LAA itself.

Device Repositioning and Retrieval

If the device is placed too distally in the appendage, it should be partially recaptured and redeployed. This is done by fixing the deployment knob and advancing the access sheath delivery system over the shoulders of the device up to but not past the distal fixation anchors. The entire system is then withdrawn to the desired location and the device redeployed by unsheathing the shoulders while fixing the deployment knob. If the device is too proximal, the operator must fully retrieve the device because it is unsafe to advance the exposed feet of the device more deeply into the LAA. After full retrieval, the delivery system is removed from the sheath, the sheath flushed, and the pigtail catheter reinserted to reposition the access sheath back into position within the LAA. The operator should identify the mechanism of implantation failure (eg, poor sheath position, inappropriate device size) and integrate this into the strategy for the next implantation attempt. A brief echocardiographic assessment for pericardial effusion should be performed after device retrieval. In the PROTECT-AF trial, the cause of pericardial effusion was thought to be the manipulation within the LAA of sheaths, wires, catheters, or the delivery system in 41% of cases, and the device deployment process in 18% of cases.[7]

Release Criteria

After the device has been implanted, TEE imaging of the LAA is performed at 0°, 45°, 90°, and 135°. Residual flow around the device, if any, should be identified. Peridevice flow greater than 5 mm is not acceptable; gaps less than or equal to 5 mm at follow-up do not seem to be associated with subsequent thromboembolic events.[16] However, it is good practice to not allow (if possible) any residual peridevice flow at the time of the procedure. Intraprocedural gaps may become bigger over time and persist, whereas new gaps can occur over time.[17] The width of the device (shoulder-to-shoulder in the plane where the threaded insert is visualized) should be measured at each angle to verify compression. The largest shoulder-to-shoulder distance should be smaller than the acceptable distance to provide adequate compression (see Table 1). Although the manufacturer recommends a compression range between 8% and 10%, many operators are more comfortable with a minimal compression greater than 10% and as high as 30%. Special attention should be paid when the device sits such that the shoulder of the device protrudes into the body of the left atrium adjacent to the mitral valve annulus and above the left atrioventricular groove (a posterior shoulder).

A large posterior shoulder can result in residual flow into the LAA if the shoulder is large enough that device's fabric cap does not cover and seal the ostium itself, and can also lead to device instability if the distal anchors along the inferoposterior circumference of the device are not interacting sufficiently with LAA tissue. Three-D TEE, color flow Doppler, left atrial angiography in the AP-caudal projection, and measurement of the distance from the widest portion of the shoulder to the LAA ostium can all provide incremental information about whether the magnitude of the posterior shoulder is acceptable.

The PASS criteria (position, anchor, size, seal) must be met before releasing the device (**Box 2**). If the PASS criteria are met, the device is released by rotating the deployment knob at the proximal end of the core wire counterclockwise. The core wire should be quickly withdrawn into the access sheath after device release so that it does not interact with, or damage, the fabric cap of the WATCHMAN.

SUMMARY

Specific technical approaches may improve the safety and efficacy of WATCHMAN LAA closure. Procedural safety is paramount because LAA closure for stroke prevention is a prophylactic procedure that is often performed in elderly patients with multiple comorbidities in whom procedural complications may not be well-tolerated. A complication rate less than 2% can be achieved with a fastidious approach that incorporates the lessons learned from early experience. Device selection can be optimized through multimodality imaging (TEE, cardiac CT, and angiography) and modest oversizing. Comprehensive TEE evaluation after implantation and before device release can identify residual leaks, large posterior shoulders, and uncovered lobes, all of which are unacceptable and may place the patient at risk for device embolism, large peridevice flow at follow-up that requires long-term OAC, and/or thromboembolic events if OAC is discontinued.

REFERENCES

1. Reddy VY, Doshi SK, Kar S, et al. 5-year outcomes after left atrial appendage closure: from the PREVAIL and PROTECT AF Trials. J Am Coll Cardiol 2017;70(24):2964–75.
2. Reddy VY, Sievert H, Halperin J, et al. Percutaneous left atrial appendage closure vs warfarin for atrial fibrillation: a randomized clinical trial. JAMA 2014; 312:1988–98.
3. Price MJ, Valderrabano M. Left atrial appendage closure to prevent stroke in patients with atrial fibrillation. Circulation 2014;130:202–12.
4. Beigel R, Wunderlich NC, Ho SY, et al. The left atrial appendage: anatomy, function, and noninvasive evaluation. JACC Cardiovasc Imaging 2014;7:1251–65.
5. Lip GY, Nieuwlaat R, Pisters R, et al. Refining clinical risk stratification for predicting stroke and thromboembolism in atrial fibrillation using a novel risk factor-based approach: the euro heart survey on atrial fibrillation. Chest 2010;137:263–72.
6. Holmes DR Jr, Kar S, Price MJ, et al. Prospective randomized evaluation of the Watchman Left Atrial Appendage Closure device in patients with atrial fibrillation versus long-term warfarin therapy: the PREVAIL trial. J Am Coll Cardiol 2014;64:1–12.
7. Reddy VY, Holmes D, Doshi SK, et al. Safety of percutaneous left atrial appendage closure: results from the Watchman Left Atrial Appendage System for Embolic Protection in Patients with AF (PROTECT AF) clinical trial and the Continued Access Registry. Circulation 2011;123:417–24.
8. Boersma LV, Schmidt B, Betts TR, et al. Implant success and safety of left atrial appendage closure with the WATCHMAN device: peri-procedural outcomes from the EWOLUTION registry. Eur Heart J 2016;37(31):2465–74
9. Holmes DR, Reddy VY, Turi ZG, et al. Percutaneous closure of the left atrial appendage versus warfarin therapy for prevention of stroke in patients with atrial fibrillation: a randomised non-inferiority trial. Lancet 2009;374:534–42.
10. DeSimone CV, Prakriti BG, Tri J, et al. A review of the relevant embryology, pathohistology, and anatomy of the left atrial appendage for the invasive

cardiac electrophysiologist. J Atr Fibrillation 2015; 8:1129.

11. Schmidt-Salzmann M, Meincke F, Kreidel F, et al. Improved algorithm for ostium size assessment in watchman left atrial appendage occlusion using three-dimensional echocardiography. J Invasive Cardiol 2017;29:232–8.

12. Wang DD, Eng M, Kupsky D, et al. Application of 3-dimensional computed tomographic image guidance to WATCHMAN implantation and impact on early operator learning curve: single-center experience. JACC Cardiovasc Interv 2016;9:2329–40.

13. Saw J, Fahmy P, Spencer R, et al. Comparing measurements of CT angiography, TEE, and fluoroscopy of the left atrial appendage for percutaneous closure. J Cardiovasc Electrophysiol 2016; 27:414–22.

14. Enomoto Y, Gadiyaram VK, Gianni C, et al. Use of non-warfarin oral anticoagulants instead of warfarin during left atrial appendage closure with the Watchman device. Heart Rhythm 2017;14:19–24.

15. Saw J, Price MJ. Assessing the safety of early U.S. Commercial application of left atrial appendage closure. J Am Coll Cardiol 2017;69:262–4.

16. Viles-Gonzalez JF, Kar S, Douglas P, et al. The clinical impact of incomplete left atrial appendage closure with the Watchman Device in patients with atrial fibrillation: a PROTECT AF (percutaneous closure of the left atrial appendage versus warfarin therapy for prevention of stroke in patients with atrial fibrillation) substudy. J Am Coll Cardiol 2012;59:923–9.

17. Bai R, Horton RP, DI Baise L, et al. Intraprocedural and long-term incomplete occlusion of the left atrial appendage following placement of the WATCHMAN device: a single center experience. J Cardiovasc Electrophysiol 2012; 23:455–61.

The Amplatzer Amulet Device
Technical Considerations and Procedural Approach

Nathan Messas, MD[a,b], Reda Ibrahim, MD[a,*]

KEYWORDS

- AMPLATZER Amulet • Left atrial appendage occlusion • Nonvalvular atrial fibrillation
- Transseptal puncture • Chicken wing anatomy

KEY POINTS

- Percutaneous left atrial appendage occlusion (LAAO) is recognized as an alternative approach to oral anticoagulation in patients with nonvalvular atrial fibrillation.
- The AMPLATZER Amulet, the second-generation device of the AMPLATZER Cardiac Plug, is currently one of the most commonly used devices for LAAO.
- Implantation of the AMPLATZER Amulet requires a step-by-step technical approach following several technical considerations.

INTRODUCTION

Percutaneous left atrial appendage occlusion (LAAO) is currently recommended as an alternative to oral anticoagulation (OAC) in patients with nonvalvular atrial fibrillation (NVAF).[1] Several devices are under clinical investigation, among which a few have already received approval. The AMPLATZER Cardiac Plug (ACP) received CE Mark in December 2008. It was the first AMPLATZER device specially designed by Dr Kurt Amplatz to close the appendage.[2] The AMPLATZER Amulet is a second-generation LAAO device. The Amulet became commercially available in Europe in January 2013 (AGA Medical, Plymouth, MN, USA acquired by St Jude Vascular, St Paul, MN, USA, followed by Abbott Vascular, Santa Clara, CA, USA).[3] In United States, the approval by the US Food and Drug Administration is still pending despite that it is one of the most widely used devices in the world.

This article reviews the key characteristics of the AMPLATZER Amulet and describes step-by-step technical considerations relevant to the implantation in the left appendage.

DEVICE DESIGN AND MAIN FEATURES OF THE AMPLATZER AMULET

The AMPLATZER Amulet is a transcatheter self-expanding device specifically designed for left atrial appendage (LAA) closure. The configuration maintains the concept and the basic structure of the original version (ACP) but was intended to improve device performance and increase safety of the device (including sealing and stability). This device consists of a distal lobe that anchors the device to the LAA body or neck (landing zone) and a proximal disc that seals the LAA orifice (ostium). Both parts of the Amulet are connected by a central waist. The main structure is made of a nitinol mesh with 2 polyester

---

Disclosure Statement: Dr N. Messas has received financial support (Fellowship grants) from Abbott Vascular France, Biotronik France, and Biosensors France. Dr R. Ibrahim is a consultant and a proctor for Abbott, Boston Scientific, Gore, and Medtronic.

[a] Department of Medicine, Montreal Heart Institute, Université de Montréal, 5000 Belanger Street, Montreal, Québec H1T 1C8, Canada; [b] Department of Cardiology, University hospital of Strasbourg, 1 place de l'hopital, Strasbourg 67000, France
* Corresponding author. Montreal Heart Institute, 5000 Belanger Street, Montreal, Québec H1T 1C8, Canada.
E-mail address: reda.ibrahim@icm-mhi.org

Intervent Cardiol Clin 7 (2018) 213–218
https://doi.org/10.1016/j.iccl.2017.12.012
2211-7458/18/© 2018 Elsevier Inc. All rights reserved.

patches sewed into both the lobe and the disc. In comparison with the ACP, the Amulet device offers the following improvements:

- A device already preloaded within the delivery system
- A wider proximal disc diameter being 6 to 7 mm greater than the distal lobe diameter (4–6 mm for the ACP)
- A thicker distal lobe length (2–3 mm thicker than the ACP)
- Stiffer stabilizing wires
- Increased number of stabilizing wires (from 6 pairs in the ACP to up to 10 pairs for the Amulet)
- Longer waist length (from 4 mm in the ACP to 5.5 mm or 8 mm depending on the size of the device)
- An inverted attaching screw on the proximal disc
- Larger sizes up to 31 and 34 mm.

LEFT ATRIAL APPENDAGE OCCLUSION CLOSURE INDICATIONS AND PROCEDURAL PLANNING

The current indications for percutaneous LAAO with the Amulet device refer to patients with NVAF requiring long-term OAC therapy.[4] Since 2012, the European Society of Cardiology implemented a class IIB recommendation for patients with high stroke risk and contraindications to long-term OAC.[1] The main contraindications for LAA closure whatever the type of device implanted are the presence of thrombus in the left atrium (which is most of the time located into the distal part of the LAA) and ongoing endocarditis or other active infectious disease.[5]

In this context, preprocedural imaging of the left atrium is warranted for each potential LAAO candidate. Investigation usually consists of performing a transesophageal echocardiography (TEE) and/or a computed tomographic (CT) scan to exclude preexisting LAA thrombus and to assess the suitability for closure, especially for sizing and device selection. Because tamponade is a potential complication of such a procedure, it is also a commendable practice to detect any preexisting pericardial effusion.

IMPLANTATION OF THE AMPLATZER AMULET DEVICE: TECHNICAL APPROACH
Intraprocedural Imaging
In terms of intraprocedural imaging, TEE is extremely helpful and is used by most operators. In that case, the procedure is typically performed under general anesthesia. Intracardiac

echography is an alternative and less-invasive option.[6] In that case, the tip of the probe can be placed in various locations but most often in the left atrium using or not the same venous access and the same transseptal puncture. This technology is well adapted to the Amplatzer given that the device is deployed in the proximal portion of the appendage. Fluoroscopy-only guided LAAO is far less optimal and should be used as a last option and by expert operators.

Real-time 3-dimensional (3D) TEE is not mandatory but is useful to provide a better spatial visualization of the anatomy. 3D is also helpful upon the final steps of the procedure notably to evaluate the stability of the occluder during the tug test and to visualize the relationship of the disc with the surrounding structures within the left atrium (using the "en face" view).

Left Atrial Appendage Occlusion Access by the Transseptal Approach
Similarly to the first generation, the AMPLATZER Amulet device is implanted through the venous system via the transseptal technique and is fully retrievable and repositionable. Like the other devices on the market, the right femoral vein is usually the preferred access site given a more direct access to the atrial septum. Transseptal puncture is then performed using a standard technique (typically using an SL1 sheath and a BRK needle; Abbott Vascular). Precision of the transseptal puncture is critical for procedural success, and the optimal site in the atrial septum is posteroinferior. A more anterior puncture is sometimes performed to reach reverse chicken wing anatomy with more anterior ostium. Of note, some operators use a patent foramen ovale or a preexisting atrial septal defect to gain access to the left atrium, thereby eliminating the need for transseptal puncture.[7] In that case, it may be acceptable to deploy an Amulet device, but in case of malalignment, a traditional transseptal approach should be done. Intravenous heparin is administered before and/or immediately following transseptal puncture to maintain an activated clotting time >250 seconds. It is also important to reach an adequate mean left atrial pressure (at least 12 mm Hg) with fluid bolus for accurate device selection.

Left Atrial Appendage Occlusion Fluoroscopic Calibration and Amulet Device Sizing
Following transseptal puncture, LAA angiograms are performed to obtain LAA measurements. For this purpose, the tip of the transseptal sheath is positioned at the level of the LAA ostium and a

5F marker pigtail is advanced into the LAA to proceed with selective injections. Cine-angiograms are performed, preferably in right anterior oblique (RAO) cranial/caudal projections. The RAO 30°–cranial 20° view is usually of interest to visualize the ostium and the neck of the appendage, whereas the RAO 30°–caudal 20° view is usually to depict better the middistal LAA anatomy (Fig. 1). The diameters of the LAA ostium and neck are then measured in both views.

Optimal device sizing is a critical step of the procedure in order to achieve complete LAA closure and avoid device embolization. Amulet sizing depends on the widest landing zone on baseline CT angiography or procedural fluoroscopy and TEE. Angiography and TEE have lower spatial resolution but have the advantage of real-time assessment during the procedure. Of note, key points for angiographic sizing are to choose the frame depicting the maximum LAA diameter and to perform a precise calibration before measurements. There is typically a good correlation (ie, <2 mm) between the different imaging modalities at corresponding points but, in case of a large discrepancy, it is important to identify which measurements are more accurate.

For sizing, a standard recommendation is to upsize the Amulet by 3 to 6 mm. This degree of oversizing should improve stability of the device and proper anchoring of the lobe. The official Amulet sizing chart refers to the maximum LAA landing zone width using 2D imaging modalities (TEE, fluoroscopy). Therefore, most operators follow this methodology. However, because the appendage is often elliptical, sizing based on the mean diameter or the perimeter of the landing zone is reasonable in cases of extreme eccentricity to avoid gross oversizing and to be sure that the lobe of the Amulet will fit into the anatomy. Conversely, slightly

more oversizing (ie, 1–2 mm more than the sizing chart recommendation) may be considered when using a small Amulet (16–22 mm), which has a shorter lobe and waist length and a lowest number of stabilizing wires in comparison with bigger sizes. Another potential reason for more oversizing is a high LAA ostium/neck ratio. In that case, a larger device disc may be needed in order to cover the LAA ostium adequately, provided there is enough space to deploy and secure the corresponding device lobe safely.

The delivery sheath size (either 12 or 14F) depends on the device size and is chosen based on a relevant chart. Oversizing of the sheath was not recommended for the ACP but is allowed for the Amulet, and some operators routinely use the larger sheath. The AMPLATZER TorqVue 45-45 sheath (Abbott Vascular) is the default sheath for both ACP and Amulet devices and has a double curve distal tip, allowing anterior and superior angulation for coaxial positioning at the landing zone.

Delivery Sheath Positioning

The next step of the procedure consists of sheath exchange and engagement of the LAA with the delivery catheter. A long (145 cm) stiff wire (eg, 0.035″ Amplatz Super Stiff J-tip 3-mm curve; Boston Scientific, Marlborough, MA, USA) is advanced through the transseptal sheath and placed in the left upper pulmonary vein. Alternatively, a long (230 cm) curve guidewire (eg, Inoue or TORAYGUIDE; Toray Medical, Chiba, Japan) can be looped in the left atrium. At this point, the use of a long 12- or 14F dilator may be considered to open well the subcutaneous tissue in the groin and to dilate the atrial septum in preparation of the exchange from the transseptal to the delivery sheath. Obese patients and tortuous

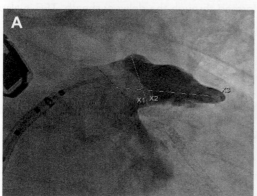 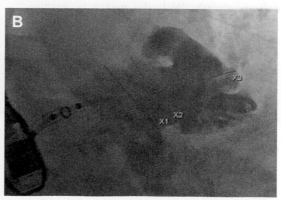

Fig. 1. LAA fluoroscopic calibration. Cine-angiograms are performed in a RAO 30°- cranial 20° (*A*) and RAO 30°- Caudal 20° (*B*) Projections. The diameters of the LAA ostium and neck are then measured in both views.

venous anatomy may also benefit from a short oversized sheath in the groin. The 12- or 14F delivery sheath (80 cm long) is then safely advanced in the left upper pulmonary vein or in the left atrium over the stiff wire. Engagement of the LAA is then performed just by pulling the delivery sheath from the left upper pulmonary vein or may be facilitate by introducing a 5- to 6F pigtail catheter or using the distal part of the Amulet device (ball shape) in front of the sheath (Fig. 2). The whole manipulation should be carried out under fluoroscopic and/or TEE guidance to ensure coaxial approach.

Device Deployment

The device introducer is carefully connected to the delivery sheath in a wet-to-wet manner opposing back-flow bleeding from the delivery sheath and forward flush through the device loader. The Y connector is slightly opened, and the device is advanced by pushing the delivery cable. Of note, it is of critical importance not to rotate the delivery cable counterclockwise to avoid disconnection of the device inside the delivery sheath. To prevent introduction of air in the system, continuous flushing from the Y-connector side arm is suggested. When the device reaches the right atrium, a quick fluoroscopic checkup is recommended to rule out air inside the sheath. At the same time, adequate connection of the device to the delivery cable is confirmed by pushing and pulling maneuvers.

Device deployment is most frequently performed in the left anterior oblique-cranial view in order to well visualize the landing zone. At this step of the procedure, the delivery catheter is gently unsheathed exposing the distal portion of the device in the so-called ball position with radiopaque markers aligned with the tip of the delivery sheath. With the device in position,

counterclockwise of the sheath is usually required to ensure a good coaxiality with the LAA landing zone. After achieving stable and optimal orientation of the sheath, the delivery cable is advanced without unsheathing to finalize distal lobe deployment. If the cable is not pushed and the operator continues to unsheath, the lobe will emerge in a more proximal position, potentially missing the landing zone. The deployment of the proximal disc is then obtained by advancing the delivery cable while unsheathing the disc (Fig. 3).

Before device release, the following 5 criteria have been defined to ensure adequate deployment:

1. An adequate compression of the distal lobe (tired shape) to LAA wall
2. A concave shape of the proximal disc for good seal
3. A separation between the distal lobe and the proximal disc
4. A distal lobe in the axis of LAA neck axis (landing zone)
5. A lobe position at least two-thirds distal to the left circumflex artery on echography.

Some operators also like to test the stability of the device by performing a gentle tug test during which the disc is put in tension (diamond shape) by pulling away from the anchored lobe. After at least 20 to 30 seconds, the tension on the delivery cable is released and the device returns to the baseline position. Finally, when an optimal device position is again confirmed, the device is released by performing counterclockwise rotations of the delivery cable.

After device deployment, TEE allows verification of the absence of peri-device leak, suggesting a good coverage of the LAA ostium. Alternatively, contrast injections can be performed through the delivery sheath. TEE is also

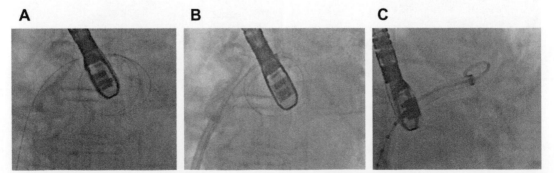

A   **B**   **C**

Fig. 2. Delivery sheath positioning. A long curve guidewire (Inoue) is looped in the left atrium (A); the delivery sheath is advanced over the Inoue wire (B). LAA engagement with the delivery sheath over a pigtail catheter (C).

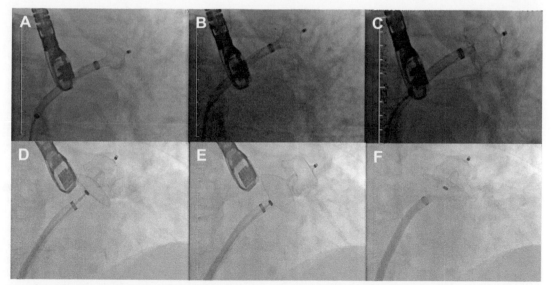

Fig. 3. Amulet deployment steps. Ball position (*A*). Counterclockwise rotation to engage the landing zone (*B*). Deployment of the distal lobe into the neck (*C*). Deployment of the proximal disc (*D*). Tug test to confirm stability (*E*). Release of the device (*F*).

useful to exclude any interference with the surrounding structures and to confirm adequate compression of the lobe of the occluder.

SPECIAL CONSIDERATIONS
Challenging Left Atrial Appendage Occlusion Morphology: The Chicken Wing Anatomy

The anatomy of the appendage is extremely variable. Some patients present with a chicken wing configuration, which is characterized by the presence of an obvious bend in the proximal or middle part of the dominant LAA lobe.[8] This anatomy can represent a challenge when the neck is very short (<15–20 mm). In that case, a sandwich technique can be considered. Its main characteristic is that the device lobe is not implanted in the standard neck position but rather parallel to the length of the LAA body (wing), resulting in sandwiching the LAA ostium between the device lobe and disc.[9] To successfully perform this technique, the delivery sheath needs to be positioned deep into the LAA using a pigtail catheter as a guide wire. Of note, the standard fluoroscopic projections may be modified in order to capture the true LAA morphology and, in most cases, a larger device is required to obtain an optimal LAA occlusion.

Patients with Refractory Left Atrial Appendage Occlusion Thrombus

The presence of an appendicular thrombus is typically a contraindication to LAAO regarding the risk of thrombus embolization. In some circumstances, an off-label percutaneous exclusion of the LAA can be considered using a no-touch technique.[10–12] In that case, the device is open partially in the left atrium to obtain a "ball shape" or a "triangular shape" that is pushed in front the thrombus to eventually form the lobe and the disc. No contrast is injected before full deployment of the device, and the delivery sheath is never advanced in the distal part of the appendage. Distal protection device in the vessels of the neck should be also considered in this instance.

SUMMARY

Recent clinical experience with the AMPLATZER Amulet has demonstrated feasibility and safety of the device for percutaneous LAAO. Novel features of the Amulet in comparison with the ACP first-generation device improve the stability of Amulet and theoretically may reduce thrombus formation on the atrial side of the device. Further investigations of the device through both observational registries and randomized trial are obviously encouraged to provide the best standard of care in patients requiring LAA closure interventions.

REFERENCES

1. Camm AJ, Lip GY, De Caterina R, et al, for the ESC Committee for Practice Guidelines. 2012 focused update of the ESC Guidelines for the management

of atrial fibrillation: an update of the 2010 ESC Guidelines for the management of atrial fibrillation. Developed with the special contribution of the European Heart Rhythm Association. Eur Heart J 2012;33:2719–47.

2. Park JW, Bethencourt A, Sievert H, et al. Left atrial appendage closure with Amplatzer cardiac plug in atrial fibrillation: initial European experience. Catheter Cardiovasc Interv 2011;77:700–6.

3. Freixa X, Abualsaud A, Chan J, et al. Left atrial appendage occlusion: initial experience with the Amplatzer™ Amulet™. Int J Cardiol 2014;174:492–6.

4. Tzikas A, Shakir S, Gafoor S, et al. Left atrial appendage occlusion for stroke prevention in atrial fibrillation: multicentre experience with the AMPLATZER cardiac plug. EuroIntervention 2016;11(10):1170–9.

5. Tzikas A, Gafoor S, Meerkin D, et al. Left atrial appendage occlusion with the AMPLATZER Amulet device: an expert consensus step-by-step approach. EuroIntervention 2016;11(13):1512–21.

6. Berti S, Paradossi U, Meucci F, et al. Periprocedural intracardiac echocardiography for left atrial appendage closure: a dual-center experience. JACC Cardiovasc Interv 2014;7(9):1036–44.

7. Koermendy D, Nietlispach F, Shakir S, et al. Amplatzer left atrial appendage occlusion through a patent foramen ovale. Catheter Cardiovasc Interv 2014;84(7):1190–6.

8. Di Biase L, Santangeli P, Anselmino M, et al. Does the left atrial appendage morphology correlate with the risk of stroke in patients with atrial fibrillation? Results from a multicenter study. J Am Coll Cardiol 2012;60:531–8.

9. Freixa X, Tzikas A, Basmadjian A, et al. The chicken-wing morphology: an anatomical challenge for left atrial appendage occlusion. J Interv Cardiol 2013; 26:509–14.

10. Aytemir K, Aminian A, Asil S, et al. First case of percutaneous left atrial appendage closure by amulet™ device in a patient with left atrial appendage thrombus. Int J Cardiol 2016;223:28–30.

11. Del Furia F, Ancona MB, Giannini F, et al. First-in-man percutaneous LAA closure with an Amplatzer Amulet and Triguard Embolic Protection Device in a patient with LAA thrombus. J Invasive Cardiol 2017;29(4):E51–2.

12. Tarantini G, D'Amico G, Latib A, et al. Percutaneous left atrial appendage occlusion in patients with atrial fibrillation and left appendage thrombus: feasibility, safety and clinical efficacy. EuroIntervention 2017. https://doi.org/10.4244/EIJ-D-17-00777.

Echocardiographic Imaging for Left Atrial Appendage Occlusion

Transesophageal Echocardiography and Intracardiac Echocardiographic Imaging

Dee Dee Wang, MD[a,*], Thomas J. Forbes, MD[b],
James C. Lee, MD[a], Marvin H. Eng, MD[a]

KEYWORDS

- Transesophageal echocardiogram • TEE • Intracardiac echocardiographic imaging • ICE • LAA

KEY POINTS

- Left atrial appendage occlusion (LAAO) is a rapidly evolving technology.
- Multi-modality imaging and understanding of left atrial appendage anatomy are sure to advance.
- Two-dimensional and 3-dimensional transesophageal echocardiography with fluoroscopy are the mainstays for LAAO image-guided therapy.
- Key to successful LAAO is an understanding of the transseptal puncture, LAAO size selection for the device-specific landing zone, and post-deployment evaluation for leak and complications.
- With advancements in computed tomography, there may be a greater role for intracardiac echocardiographic imaging in specific types of LAAO anatomy and devices.

By imaging, the left atrial appendage (LAA) is the most-neglected and least understood anatomic structure of the heart. The LAA is chronically oversimplified as a blind-ending pouch projecting off of the left lateral wall of the left atrium.[1] Its importance was not appreciated until the LAA was deemed responsible for approximately 90% of cerebral thromboembolic events in the setting of nonvalvular atrial fibrillation.[1] Before the advent of percutaneous LAA occlusion therapies, traditional outpatient LAA imaging focused purely on the presence or absence of thrombus formation in the appendage before an electrophysiology ablation or cardioversion procedure for atrial fibrillation. However, recent advancements in endovascular LAA occlusion (LAAO) devices has necessitated a deeper understanding of the LAA anatomy.

LAAO interventions are not benign procedures.[2,3] In the PROTECT AF (Watchman Left Atrial Appendage System for Embolic Protection in Patients With Atrial Fibrillation) early clinical trial, new WATCHMAN (Boston Scientific, Natick, Massachusetts) implanters carried a 5% to 7% risk of LAA closure-related complications secondary to early operator learning curve associated with limited understanding of device deployment and sizing of the LAA.

[a] Center for Structural Heart Disease, Henry Ford Hospital, 2799 West Grand Boulevard, Clara Ford Pavilion 4th Floor, Detroit, MI 48202, USA; [b] Carmen and Ann Adams Department of Pediatrics, Children's Hospital of Michigan, Pediatric Cardiology, Wayne State University School of Medicine, 3901 Beaubien Street, Detroit, MI 48202, USA
* Corresponding author.
E-mail address: DWANG2@hfhs.org

Intervent Cardiol Clin 7 (2018) 219–228
https://doi.org/10.1016/j.iccl.2018.01.001
2211-7458/18/© 2018 Elsevier Inc. All rights reserved.

In the United States, WATCHMAN is currently the only commercially available endoluminal device available for LAAO. In US clinical trials, there is a second device under investigation, named the Amplatzer AMULET (Abbott Corp, Saint Paul, Minnesota). Both devices are commercially available in Europe. Competing markets and vastly different LAAO device shapes and anchoring mechanisms has led to increased understanding of the complexity and varied morphology of the LAA.[4] With more than one device size and shape option available, more emphasis is placed on periprocedural imaging evaluation of the LAA to optimize patient-specific device selection.

Present-day LAAO procedural evaluations have been done using transesophageal echocardiography (TEE) imaging. At this time, most implanters routinely use TEE imaging to assess LAA device size selection, residual shunting, and final device placement.[5] However, some operators have developed comfort in using intracardiac echocardiographic imaging (ICE) for LAAO. This article focuses on the application of key periprocedural imaging steps necessary for successful LAAO and techniques to use TEE and ICE for LAAO.

UNDERSTANDING LANDMARKS AND IMPACT TO LEFT ATRIAL APPENDAGE OCCLUSION

Imaging for LAA intervention requires knowledge of the chosen device, potential device-specific procedural complications, and patient-specific LAA anatomy.

The endocardial surface of the LAA has a complex trabeculated structure with a variable degree of pectinate muscles.[6] Crevices between pectinate muscles are potential areas for thrombus formation. Trabeculations within the LAA may limit the ability of devices to fully expand to their maximal width within the LAA landing zone.

The body of the LAA typically lies immediately anterior and inferior to the left upper pulmonary vein (LUPV) (Fig. 1). The separation between the LAA and the LUPV is commonly

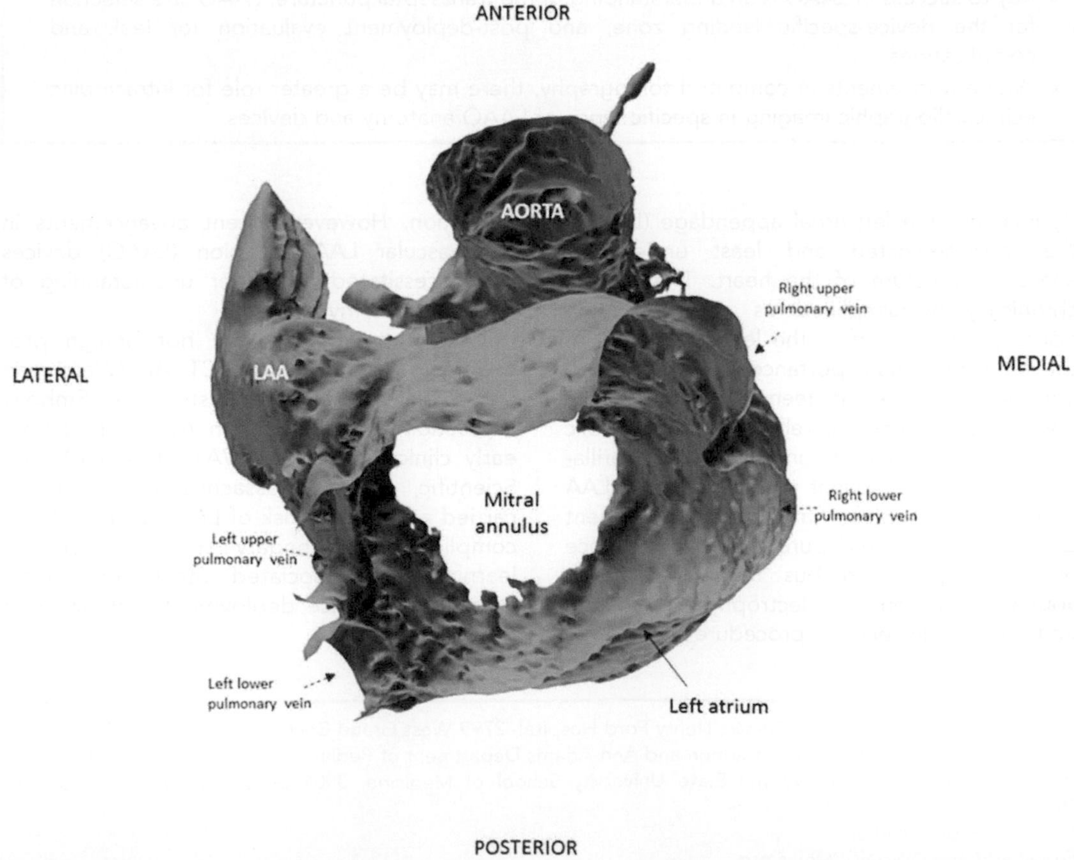

Fig. 1. Surgeon's view of the left atrium and LAA. An anatomy overview of the surrounding anatomic structures influencing the shape and landmarks for device implantation.

referred to as the lateral ridge, or Coumadin ridge, one of the early sites for detection of pericardial effusion from LAA perforation.

The LAA overlies several important structures. Landmarks include proximal left circumflex coronary artery and the great cardiac vein. The proximity of these structures is important to note, as an oversized device in the LAA may cause compression of these nearby vessels. The mitral annulus is immediately inferior to the ostium of the LAA (Fig. 2). With larger devices, care must be taken to interrogate the function of the mitral valve before and after LAAO to ensure no impingement of valve leaflets has occurred.

Fluid status is equally important in assessing the size of the LAA anatomy. Intraprocedural volume loading under transseptal guidance demonstrates the LAA to be a pliant structure. Dynamic infusion of 500 to 1000 mL of fluid can increase the LAA orifice dimension by approximately 9% and the depth by approximately 6%, thereby affecting the potential device size and selection.[7] Additionally, the volumetric size of the LAA varies between atrial fibrillation and normal sinus rhythm. The LAA is notably larger in atrial fibrillation (7060 mm^3 as compared with 4645 mm^3 in sinus rhythm, P<.01).[6]

Knowledge of LAA anatomy and its surrounding structures is critical to the success of LAAO.

INTRAPROCEDURAL IMAGING-GUIDED THERAPY

Key Steps to Successful Left Atrial Appendage Occlusion via Transesophageal Echocardiography

Room setup
For optimal TEE-guided intervention, it is essential for the TEE operator to have visual access to a real-time fluoroscopic monitor display (Fig. 3). This access allows the imaging operator to keep an eye on fluoroscopic catheter movements while simultaneously correlating the TEE images to catheter adjustments to prevent miscommunication.

Transseptal puncture
In most patients without a hiatal hernia, or congenital anatomic defects of the heart, the fossa ovalis is located superior and posterior to the orifice of the LAA (Fig. 4). Hence, the optimal site of transseptal puncture is an inferior and posterior crossing on the fossa ovalis. A well-executed transseptal puncture can make a significant difference in the LAA procedure duration and ease of device positioning.

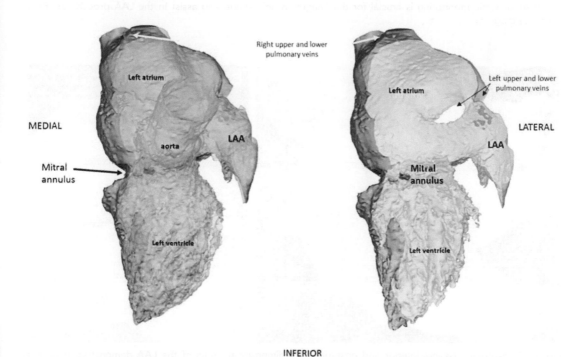

Fig. 2. Two-chamber view of the LAA. From a medial to lateral cross-sectional analysis of the LAA, all surrounding anatomic landmarks can be better appreciated for optimal device visualization and impact to adjacent structures.

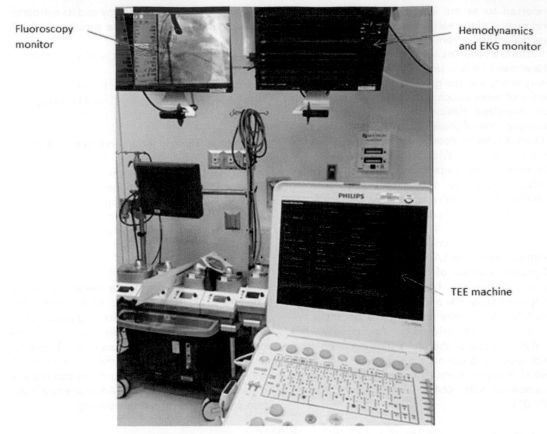

Fig. 3. Recommended room setup for the Interventional Imager. Access to real-time fluoroscopic imaging displays and hemodynamic monitoring is crucial for the Imager to help guide and assist in the LAA procedures. EKG, electrocardiogram.

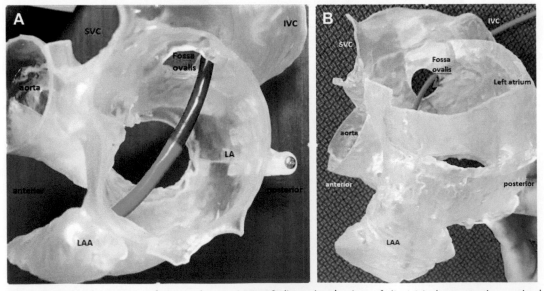

Fig. 4. Transseptal crossing. Inferior and posterior on 3-dimensional prints of the LAA demonstrating optimal crossing point from multiple angulations (A, B) of the surgeon's view of the left atrium. IVC, inferior vena cava; LA, left atrium; SVC, superior vena cava.

Optimal image guidance for transseptal crossing includes visualization of the fossa ovalis in the midesophageal short-axis aortic valve view on TEE, with a simultaneous 90° biplane (Fig. 5) view of the septum reflected next to it. This image would project the anterior and posterior rims (Fig. 6) of the fossa ovalis on the left panel and the superior and inferior rims of the fossa ovalis on the right panel (Fig. 7).

Screening and sizing the left atrial appendage landing zone. Periprocedural imaging of the LAA is important for the detection of potential sources of embolism before LAAO and for device sizing.[1] If intracardiac mass or thrombus is suspected within the left atrium (LA) or the LAA, echocardiographic contrast can be administered to help delineate between pectinate muscles, artifact, or thrombus.

Sizing for LAAO depends on the type of device selected for patient-specific implantation. At baseline, the LAA is imaged at the midesophageal to high-esophageal levels to allow maximal visualization of the LAA landing zone. Standard multiplane measurements are obtained at 0°, 45°, 90°, and 135° views on 2-dimensional (2D) TEE imaging (Fig. 8). Careful rotation and manipulation of the TEE probe should be performed dynamically at each angulation to ensure all potential lobes of the LAA are visualized.[1] Optimally, 3-dimensional (3D) TEE imaging of the LAA should also be obtained to allow an on phos (or direct 3D) visualization of the LAA opening to account for ellipsoid landing shapes that may be missed on traditional 2D TEE images. For the AMULET device, the maximal LAA diameter taken at these angulations at a depth of 10 to 15 mm from the ostium is used in device size selection.[8] For the WATCHMAN

device implant, the maximal diameter and depth of the LAA at each angulation taken at the level of the course of the circumflex artery approximately 1 to 2 cm inferior to the limbus of the Coumadin ridge is obtained in device size selection. In the WATCHMAN implantation, the depth from the landing zone of the device to the distal tip of the LAA should exceed the maximal diameter of the device size selected to prevent the risk of LAA perforation during deployment.

Postdeployment evaluation and surveillance. After implantation of the LAAO device, imaging should again be performed at the mid to high esophageal levels to evaluate device stability, anchoring, and peri-device leak. Given the low-flow state in the LAA, the Nyquist limit should be set to less than 40 cm/s when interrogating for a peri-device leak. For the WATCHMAN implantation, maximal device diameter measurements again need to be taken at the standard angulation views to account for sufficient device size compression before release of the LAAO device. Before removal of the TEE probe, a final deep transgastric evaluation of the pericardium should be performed to ensure there is no evidence of pericardial effusion after LAAO. On 45-day imaging follow-up, care should be taken to evaluate the 0°, 45°, 90°, and 135° views both with and without color to evaluate for peri-device leak and the presence or absence of intracardiac or device surface thrombus.

Role of Intracardiac Echocardiographic Imaging in Left Atrial Appendage Occlusion

The important aspect of using ICE imaging for LAA closure procedures, similar to using ICE

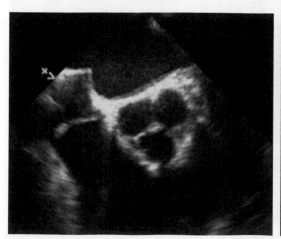
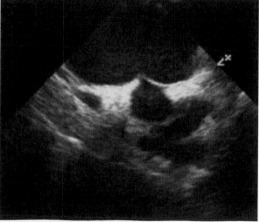

Fig. 5. Biplane view of the interatrial septum for guiding transseptal crossing.

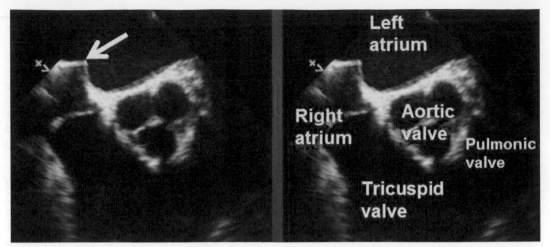

Fig. 6. Anterior posterior view of the interatrial septum and accompanying landmarks for guiding transseptal puncture. The arrow is pointing to the transseptal needle tenting the interatrial septum right before crossing into the left atrium.

imaging in closing atrial septal defects, is to not attempt to duplicate TEE images but treat it as an entirely different imaging modality. The main advantage of using TEE to image the LAA for closure relates to the omni-plane imaging capabilities of TEE, whereby views ranging from 0° to 180° can be routinely obtained. In contrast, the two currently available ICE imaging catheters, AcuNav (Biosense-Webster, Diamond Bar, California) and the ViewFlex PLUS (Abbott Medical, Minneapolis, Minnesota), are phased array catheters with 64 elements used to scan in a 90° longitudinal monoplane at frequencies ranging from 4.5 to 10.0 MHz. Both catheters are able

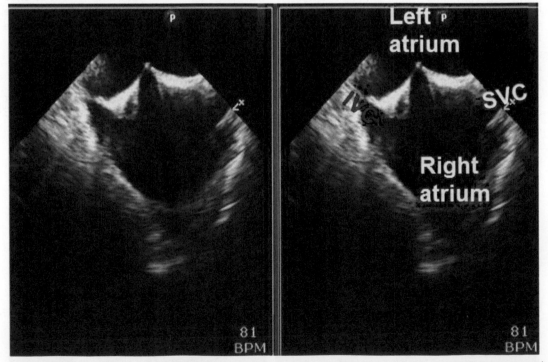

Fig. 7. Superior and inferior view of the interatrial septum and accompanying landmarks for guiding transseptal puncture. IVC, inferior vena cava; SVC, superior vena cava.

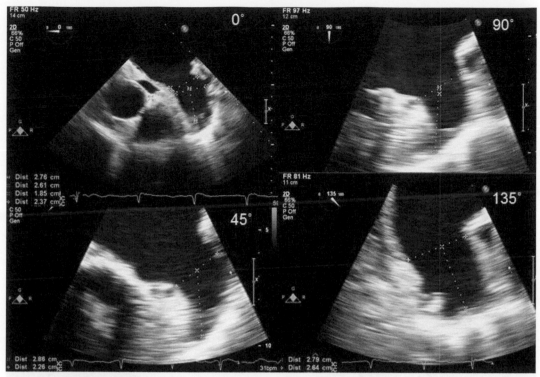

Fig. 8. Standard 2D 0°, 45°, 90°, and 135° views of the LAA.

to move in all 4 planes. Because of the monoplane imaging characteristics, proper imaging using ICE catheters requires manipulation of the catheter by the operator.

The first reported use of ICE imaging was to assist in transseptal crossing for left-sided interventions toward closing interatrial communications.[9,10] Since the first report of using ICE to assist in closure of LAA by Ho and colleagues[11] in 2007, more institutions have been reporting their experience in using ICE as a potential imaging modality to replace TEE.[5,12,13] The use of ICE is slowly gaining acceptance in Europe, with it just gaining traction in the United States for LAAO.

Intracardiac Echocardiographic Imaging Techniques

There are 2 ways one can image the LAA to assist in LAA closure procedures using ICE. The first one is to perform right-sided imaging.

There are 3 areas one can attempt to image the LAA from the right side. The easiest, but least reliable, way to image the LAA is from the right atrium (RA) (Fig. 9). Adequate imaging can be obtained in most patients using this method; however, there are several limitations to this technique. When using the 8F ICE imaging probe, the distance from the RA to the

LAA may be beyond the depth of the field. Furthermore, depending on the orientation of the LAA, oblique views of the LAA for assessment of peri-device leaks are frequently not obtainable. A second method is to introduce the ICE catheter into the distal coronary sinus (CS). In contrast to RA probe placement for LAA imaging, CS positioning allows for more optimal long axis, ostial, and landing zone LAA dimensions. Consistent oblique views of the LAA are frequently not obtainable because of the limitations of probe movement within the restrictive CS. In spite of this, Berti and colleagues[14] showed that in 51 consecutive patients, ICE imaging from the right side (RA and/or the CS) showed good correlation to both TEE and angiography regarding overall LAA anatomy and ostial/landing zone dimensions. However, all of these patients did undergo preprocedural TEE; these measurements were relied on heavily for device size selection.[14] Additionally, the AMULET device was implanted and not the WATCHMAN. Hence, commentation on interrogation for peri-device leak after the LAAO is limited, as this is not performed in multi-planar angles for the AMULET protocol.

The final right-sided imaging method of the LAA is placement of the ICE catheter in the right ventricular outflow tract (RVOT) toward the

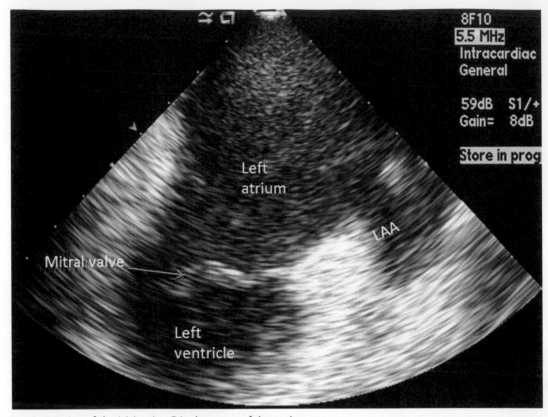

Fig. 9. Imaging of the LAA using RA placement of the probe.

distal main pulmonary artery/proximal pulmonary artery junction. Given the stiffness of the ICE catheter, the risks to this technique include potential trauma to the RVOT through manipulation of the catheter. In each of these methods, fine manipulations of probe placement in the RVOT will allow for long-axis views of the LAA. Further advancement of the probe to the proximal left pulmonary artery gives an oblique view of the LAA. Advancing the ICE catheter across the RVOT allows for more consistent imaging of peri-device leaks.

The most reliable approach to imaging the LAA using ICE is to directly place the catheter into the LA proper. The ICE catheter is introduced into the LA either through a separate transseptal puncture, through double wiring a sheath, or, in some cases, just advancing the ICE catheter next to the wire placed through the initial transseptal puncture procedure.[12] One can duplicate TEE imaging from 0° to 120° with the ICE catheter being directly placed into the LA (Fig. 10). The catheter is first positioned at the left upper pulmonary vein (see Fig. 10A). This location gives a long-axis view of the LAA and device placement (see

Fig. 10B, C). Withdrawal of the catheter toward the right side of the LA and slightly inferiorly allows for oblique imaging of the LAA (see Fig. 10D) for peri-device leaks.

Placement of the ICE catheter directly into the LA to obtain LAA images most closely correlates to both computed tomography (CT) and TEE sizing of the LAA.[14,15] The largest series to date by Korsholm, and colleagues[15] noted that ICE imaging of the LAA showed good correlation with TEE measurements and device procedural success. At follow-up TEE imaging, peri-device leaks were similar to standard TEE imaging, with 96.1% noting less than 3-mm leaks and 3.9% between 3- and 5-mm leaks. However, this study relied heavily on preprocedural CT imaging of the LAA anatomy in device size selection. Again, the AMULET device was exclusively used. This combination of CT preprocedural planning and intraprocedural ICE guidance for AMULET implantation suggests a potential decreased incidence of peri-device leaks.[15]

Placement of the ICE catheter directly into the LA is comparable with the standard 45° or 90° TEE imaging planes. With advancements in preprocedural CT in LAAO sizing and patient

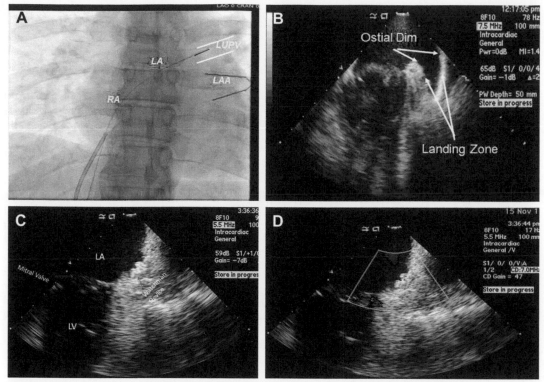

Fig. 10. Fluoroscopic landmarks and intracardiac echocardiographic imaging pre- and post-WATCHMAN device implantation. (*A*) The ICE catheter is first positioned at the left upper pulmonary vein. Dual white lines project the outline of the left upper pulmonary vein (LUPV) on fluoroscopy. The red line demonstrates the outline of the LAA. (*B, C*) ICE imaging of the LAA pre and post WATCHMAN implantation. Color flow imaging of the LAA (*D*) demonstrating no peridevice leaks. LA, left atrium; LUPV, left upper pulmonary vein; LV, left ventricle; RA, right atrium.

device selection, there is a potential role for ICE to guide intraprocedural imaging for specific LAA variations without the need for intraprocedural TEE oversight.

SUMMARY

LAAO is a rapidly evolving technology. Multimodality imaging and understanding of LAA anatomy are sure to advance. Two-dimensional and 3D TEE with fluoroscopy are the mainstays for LAAO image-guided therapy. Key to successful LAAO is an understanding of the transseptal puncture, LAAO size selection for the device-specific landing zone, and postdeployment evaluation for leaks and complications. With advancements in CT, there may be a greater role for ICE in specific types of LAAO anatomy and devices.

REFERENCES

1. Wunderlich NC, Beigel R, Swaans MJ, et al. Percutaneous interventions for left atrial appendage exclusion: options, assessment, and imaging using 2D and 3D echocardiography. JACC Cardiovasc Imaging 2015;8(4):472–88.

2. Reddy VY, Holmes D, Doshi SK, et al. Safety of percutaneous left atrial appendage closure: results from the Watchman left atrial appendage system for embolic protection in patients with AF (PROTECT AF) clinical trial and the continued access registry. Circulation 2011; 123(4):417–24.

3. Holmes DR, Kar S, Price MJ Jr, et al. Prospective randomized evaluation of the watchman left atrial appendage closure device in patients with atrial fibrillation versus long-term warfarin therapy: the PREVAIL trial. J Am Coll Cardiol 2014;64(1):1–12.

4. Wang Y, Di Biase L, Horton RP, et al. Left atrial appendage studied by computed tomography to help planning for appendage closure device placement. J Cardiovasc Electrophysiol 2010;21(9): 973–82.

5. Matsuo Y, Neuzil P, Petru J, et al. Left atrial appendage closure under intracardiac echocardiographic guidance: feasibility and comparison with

transesophageal echocardiography. J Am Heart Assoc 2016;5(10) [pii: e003695].

6. Ernst G, Stöllberger C, Abzieher F, et al. Morphology of the left atrial appendage. Anat Rec 1995;242(4):553–61.

7. Spencer RJ, DeJong P, Fahmy P, et al. Changes in left atrial appendage dimensions following volume loading during percutaneous left atrial appendage closure. JACC Cardiovasc Interv 2015;8(15):1935–41.

8. Abualsaud A, Freixa X, Tzikas A, et al. Side-by-side comparison of LAA occlusion performance with the Amplatzer cardiac plug and Amplatzer amulet. J Invasive Cardiol 2016;28(1):34–8.

9. Daoud EG, Kalbfleisch SJ, Hummel JD. Intracardiac echocardiography to guide transseptal left heart catheterization for radiofrequency catheter ablation. J Cardiovasc Electrophysiol 1999;10(3): 358–63.

10. Hijazi Z, Wang Z, Cao Q, et al. Transcatheter closure of atrial septal defects and patent foramen ovale under intracardiac echocardiographic guidance: feasibility and comparison

with transesophageal echocardiography. Catheter Cardiovasc Interv 2001;52(2):194–9.

11. Ho IC, Neuzil P, Mraz T, et al. Use of intracardiac echocardiography to guide implantation of a left atrial appendage occlusion device (PLAATO). Heart Rhythm 2007;4(5):567–71.

12. Aguirre D, Pincetti C, Perez L, et al. Single trans-septal access technique for left atrial intracardiac echocardiography to guide left atrial appendage closure. Catheter Cardiovasc Interv 2018;91(2):356–61.

13. Masson JB, Kouz R, Riahi M, et al. Transcatheter left atrial appendage closure using intracardiac echocardiographic guidance from the left atrium. Can J Cardiol 2015;31(12):1497.e7–14.

14. Berti S, Paradossi U, Meucci F, et al. Periprocedural intracardiac echocardiography for left atrial appendage closure: a dual-center experience. JACC Cardiovasc Interv 2014;7(9):1036–44.

15. Korsholm K, Jensen JM, Nielsen-Kudsk JE. Intracardiac echocardiography from the left atrium for procedural guidance of transcatheter left atrial appendage occlusion. JACC Cardiovasc Interv 2017;10(21):2198–206.

Cardiac Computed Tomography for Left Atrial Appendage Occlusion
Acquisition, Analysis, Advantages, and Limitations

Kasper Korsholm, MD, Jesper Møller Jensen, MD, PhD,
Jens Erik Nielsen-Kudsk, MD, DMSc*

KEYWORDS

- Left atrial appendage occlusion • Cardiac computed tomography • Device sizing
- Left atrial appendage thrombus • Peridevice leaks

KEY POINTS

- Transcatheter left atrial appendage occlusion is a challenging procedure, which requires accurate imaging to appreciate the highly variable anatomy of the left atrial appendage.
- Cardiac computed tomography (CT) offers high-resolution 3-dimensional imaging, which may be a viable alternative to transesophageal echocardiography for screening, planning, and postimplant device surveillance of left atrial appendage occlusion.
- Important functions of cardiac CT are left atrial appendage thrombus exclusion, assessment of suitable anatomies for implantation, and device sizing, along with postprocedural evaluation of residual peridevice leakage, and device-related thrombosis.

 Video content accompanies this article at http://www.interventional.theclinics.com

INTRODUCTION

Transcatheter left atrial appendage occlusion (LAAO) is increasingly used for stroke prevention in atrial fibrillation (AF). More than 90% of thrombi in patients with nonvalvular AF originate from the left atrial appendage (LAA).[1] Thereby, providing the rationale for LAAO as an alternative to oral anticoagulation. The Watchman (Boston Scientific, Marlborough, MA, USA), and the Amplatzer Cardiac Plug (ACP) and Amulet (Abbott, Lake Bluff, IL, USA) are the most widely used endocardial occluder devices. Two randomized trials[2,3] and multiple observational registries[4–7] have proven the efficacy and safety of these devices. In turn, the 2016 European Society of Cardiology guidelines on AF recommend considering LAAO in patients with previous major bleeding and contraindication to oral anticoagulation (Class IIb).[8]

LAAO is technically challenging because of the complex anatomy of the LAA. Thus, imaging is paramount to performing a successful LAAO. Transesophageal echocardiography (TEE) is considered the gold standard for imaging of the LAA.[9] However, cardiac computed tomography (CT) is increasingly used as a viable

---

Conflict of Interest: K. Korsholm has received speaker's honorarium and a traveling grant from Abbott; J.M. Jensen has received speaker's honorarium from Bracco Imaging, and J.E. Nielsen-Kudsk is a proctor for Abbott.
Department of Cardiology, Aarhus University Hospital, Palle Juul-Jensens Boulevard 99, Aarhus N DK-8200, Denmark
* Corresponding author.
E-mail address: je.nielsen.kudsk@gmail.com

Intervent Cardiol Clin 7 (2018) 229–242
https://doi.org/10.1016/j.iccl.2017.12.004
2211-7458/18/© 2017 Elsevier Inc. All rights reserved.

alternative in both preprocedural planning and postprocedural device surveillance. The noninvasive 3-dimensional (3D) multiplanar capability, with high spatial resolution, makes it ideal for visualizing complex anatomic structures, such as the LAA. Herein, the authors review the practical utility of cardiac CT in the setting of LAAO.

CARDIAC COMPUTED TOMOGRAPHY FOR ANATOMIC CHARACTERIZATION OF THE LEFT ATRIAL APPENDAGE

The LAA varies considerably in size, shape, and spatial relations.[10–12] Through volume-rendering technique and 3D multiplanar reconstructed cardiac CT, a careful anatomic

characterization is made possible. Most commonly, the LAA extends as a fingerlike projection between the anterior and lateral wall of the left atrium, with its tip directed anterolateral in close proximity to the right ventricular outflow tract and pulmonary trunk[12–15] (Fig. 1A, B). Morphologic classification of the LAA can be performed using 3D volume-rendered cardiac CT (Fig. 2). The most widely used CT classification consists of 4 distinct shapes[14,16]: the *chicken wing*, characterized by a distinct proximal bend of the dominant lobe; the *windsock*, with a dominant lobe and secondary lobes arising in the inferior direction; the *cactus*, consisting of a dominant central lobe with secondary lobes arising in both the superior and the inferior

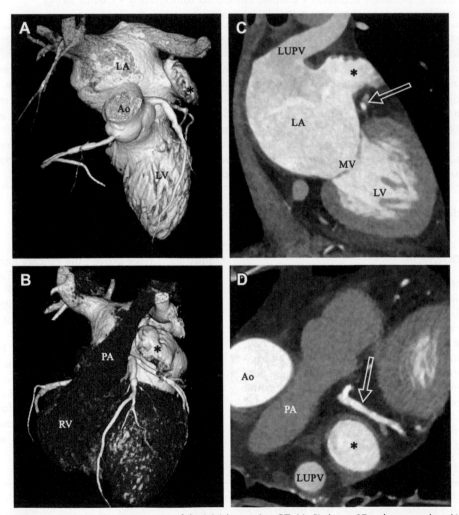

Fig. 1. Anatomy and surrounding structures of the LAA by cardiac CT. (*A, B*) shows 3D volume-rendered images of the heart with and without the right ventricle and pulmonary artery visualized in relation to the LAA (*asterisk*). (*C*) Coronal view (right anterior oblique 30°, cranial 10°) of the LAAO with surrounding anatomy. The arrow marks the circumflex coronary artery. (*D*) Axial en face view of the LAAO with surrounding anatomic structures. Ao, aorta; LA, left atrium; LV, left ventricle; LUPV, left upper pulmonary vein; MV, mitral valve; PA, pulmonary artery; RV, right ventricle. The *asterisk* demarcate the left atrial appendage and the *arrow* marks the circumflex coronary artery.

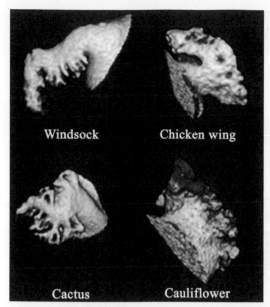

Fig. 2. 3D cardiac CT-derived morphologies of the LAA.

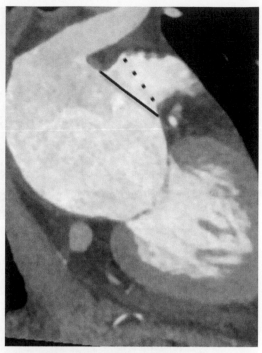

Fig. 3. Anatomic and echocardiographic orifice. The dashed line shows the anatomic orifice of the LAA, connecting the circumflex coronary artery inferior to a point 1 to 2 cm inside the LAA from the pulmonary vein ridge. The solid line shows the echocardiographic orifice, demarcated by the circumflex coronary artery and the tip of the left upper pulmonary vein ridge.

direction; whereas the *cauliflower* is short, with a broad base without a dominant lobe, but characterized by several lobes and complex internal trabeculation close to the orifice (see **Fig. 2**). The chicken wing morphology is most common, with cauliflower being least common.[13,14,16,17] Different morphologies may be associated with different risks of thromboembolism, with the chicken wing being associated with the lowest risk.[17] However, the chicken wing morphology constitutes a particular challenge when performing LAAO.[18,19]

Through multiplanar reconstructed views, the LAA orifice can be visualized between the mitral valve inferiorly, and the left pulmonary veins superiorly and posteriorly.[10,12] The circumflex coronary artery can be depicted in the atrioventricular groove[10] (**Fig. 1C**). For interventional purposes, it is relevant to distinguish between the echocardiographic and anatomic orifice.[20] The echocardiographic orifice is defined as a line connecting the circumflex coronary artery inferiorly with the tip of the pulmonary vein ridge at the superior junction of the orifice (**Fig. 3**).[12] The anatomic orifice is defined as the junction between the smooth-walled left atrium and the trabeculated LAA, represented by a line connecting the circumflex coronary artery inferiorly and a point 1 to 2 cm within the pulmonary vein ridge (see **Fig. 3**).[12] Multiplanar cross-sectional views of the orifice can assist when defining the shape of the orifice (**Fig. 4**).[14]

LEFT ATRIAL APPENDAGE THROMBUS AND CARDIAC COMPUTED TOMOGRAPHIC TECHNIQUES

The diagnostic accuracy of multidetector cardiac CT to detect and exclude LAA thrombus has been extensively investigated. One of the major difficulties with cardiac CT is differentiation between contrast filling defects (LAA stasis) and LAA thrombus[21] (**Fig. 5**). Sensitivity of cardiac CT to detect LAA thrombus is reported between 29% and 100% with a specificity of 67% to 100%, and positive predictive value (PPV) of 12% to 100%.[21–29] A recent meta-analysis of 19 studies showed a mean sensitivity of 96% and specificity of 92%.[28] However, the most consistent finding was a high negative predictive value (NPV) ranging between 96% and 100% across studies.[28] As a consequence, most investigators conclude that patients without filling defects on cardiac CT do not require additional TEE examination.

Cardiac CT protocol modifications have been suggested to increase the specificity. Most widely used is delayed image acquisition, with

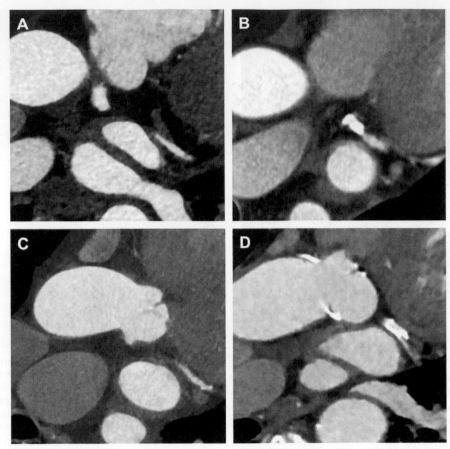

Fig. 4. Shapes of the LAAO. Four different cardiac CT-derived shapes of the LAAO. (*A*) A foot-shaped orifice; (*B*) round orifice; (*C*) oval-shaped orifice; (*D*) water-drop shaped orifice.

a second scan performed 30 to 180 seconds after the initial scan. Thereby, both filling defects and LAA thrombus should be visible in the early phase images, whereas only the LAA thrombus persists on the delayed images. The reported increase in accuracy appears consistent, with specificity ranging between 98% and 100% and PPV between 79% and 100%, whereas sensitivity and NPV remain 100%.[25,28–30] However, the associated increase in radiation may be a matter of concern. An alternative proposal is dual-enhancement, involving 2 separate contrast injections with delayed administration, followed by a single-phase scan.[26,27,31] The differentiation between filling defects and thrombus is subsequently evaluated by contrast attenuation and shape. LAA thrombus appears round or oval in shape, whereas filling defects appear triangular with homogenous signal intensity.[26,27] However, the dual-enhancement technique may constitute a problem in patients with renal impairment, because of the nearly doubled contrast exposure.

In addition to the visual (qualitative) assessment for LAA thrombus, a quantitative approach has been investigated.[23,25–27,32,33] The Hounsfield unit ratio between the LAA and ascending aorta is the most frequently used. Although a consistently lower Hounsfield unit ratio for thrombus than filling defects has been reported, the cutoff values vary greatly between studies.[23,25–27,32,33] In addition, the use of the Hounsfield unit ratio has been reported to worsen the diagnostic performance as compared with the visual assessment.[27,32,34,35] A promising alternative is assessment of iodine concentration using the newer-generation dual-energy source scanners. However, data are limited and require further validation.[34]

CARDIAC COMPUTED TOMOGRAPHIC ACQUISITION FOR LEFT ATRIAL APPENDAGE OCCLUSION

Different imaging protocols and scanners have been used in the literature for acquisition before

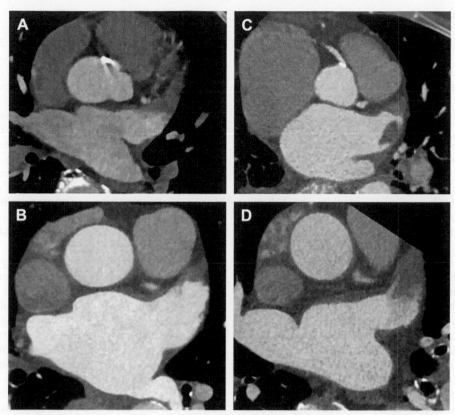

Fig. 5. Cardiac CT evaluation for LAA thrombus. (A) Large contrast filling defect, with irregular surface. (B) Small distal contrast filling defect representing incomplete contrast mixing. (C) Two distinct filling defects with convex or concave shape representing LAA thrombus. (D) Large filling defect, with a clearly delineated thrombus with signs of reduced contrast mixing proximal to the thrombus.

and after LAAO. Single- and dual-source scanners seem equally used.[36–43] All studies use electrocardiographic triggering, with prospective gating and dose modulation in the majority.[36,40–43] Both test bolus and automated bolus tracking techniques are applied, with no uniform Hounsfield unit threshold (80–130 HU),[39,42,44] and the region of interest varies between the left atrium,[39] left ventricle,[41] and ascending aorta.[42] Slice thickness is between 0.5 and 0.75 mm, with image reconstruction at ~30% to 40% or ~75% to 85% of R-R interval, depending on the heart rate.[36,37,39–41,43,45] One study describes using beta-blockers if heart rates are greater than 65 beats per minute.[41]

At the authors' institution, both 128- and 196-dual source scanners have been used (Siemens SOMATOM Definition Flash or SOMATOM Force scanners; Siemens, Forchheim, Germany). A topogram scan is performed to localize the heart, and a 10-mL test bolus of contrast (Iomerone, Bracco Imaging, Milan, Italy or Optiray, Mallinckrodt Pharmaceuticals, Staines-upon-Thames, United Kingdom, 350 mg/mL)

for assessment of peak enhancement in the LAA and ascending aorta. Datasets are acquired using prospective electrocardiographic triggering, with a high-pitch single-heart-beat spiral acquisition (Turbo FLASH) under breath hold. The scan is targeting a diastolic phase for heart rates less than 70 beats per minute, and a systolic phase for heart rates ≥70 beats per minute. Tube voltage is between 70 and 150 kV depending on body weight. Automated tube current modulation is used (CareDose 4D, Siemens), with a gantry rotation time of 0.25 seconds and collimation of 2 × 196 × 0.75 mm. A single contrast bolus (40–60 mL, Iomerone or Optiray 350 mg I/mL) is administered through an antecubital vein at a flow rate of 5 to 6 mL/s, followed by a 50 mL saline flush. Contrast dosage is adjusted according to renal function and body weight. Images are reconstructed at ~65% of R-R interval for heart rates less than 70 beats per minute, using an iterative model reconstruction and a kernel Bv40. In the event of rapid heart rates, a systole reconstruction (~40% R-R interval) is preferred. Sublingual nitroglycerin

0.8 mg is administered to all patients in order to visualize the circumflex coronary artery. No beta-blocker administration is used. The same scan protocol is used for preprocedural and postprocedural imaging. A step-by-step approach is provided in **Fig. 6** and **Table 1**.

RADIATION EXPOSURE

The associated radiation exposure varies depending on the type of scanner and acquisition protocol. For 64-slice scanners, a mean effective radiation dosage of 18.1 ± 5.9 mSv has been described.[41] Radiation exposure for 128-slice dual-source scanners has been reported in the range of 1.9 to 5.2 mSv, with a median of 3.5 mSv.[36,42] Similarly, a mean radiation exposure for 320-slice scanners has been reported as 3.9 ± 1.8 mSv.[41,44] In a study with combined use of 128-dual source and 320-single source scanners, the mean radiation exposure was 6.6 ± 4.5 mSv.[46] Prospective electrocardiographic gating, tube current modulation, high-pitch scanning mode, and iterative reconstruction technique can reduce radiation exposure.[47–49]

The mean radiation dose associated with other cardiac procedures, such as diagnostic coronary angiography, has been reported as 8.1 ± 6.4 mSv,[50] and 4 mSv (1.4–17) in regular pacemaker or implantable cardioverter defibrillator implantation.[51]

ANALYSIS OF PREPROCEDURAL CARDIAC COMPUTED TOMOGRAPHY FOR FEASIBILITY AND DEVICE SIZING

A wide range of imaging processing workstations are available, such as the syngo.via (Siemens Healthcare, Erlangen, Germany), Vitrea (Toshiba Medical Systems Group Co, Zoetermeer, Netherlands), Brilliance (Philips Healthcare, Eindhoven, The Netherlands), 3mensio software (Pie Medical Imaging, Bilthoven, The Netherlands), and OsiriX software (Pixmeo SARL, Bernex, Switzerland). These allow automated 3D multiplanar reconstructions based on conventional axial images. The software allows the user to assess the LAA and surrounding structures manually in multiple planes, thus, among others enabling selection of the optimal fluoroscopic angulations for procedural guidance. Some software packages even provide fluoroscopic simulations of the anatomy. Thus enabling the operator to precisely characterize anatomic structures relevant to the LAAO and to plan the procedural steps.

The geometric shape and morphology of the LAA can be visualized by volume-rendered 3D reconstructions, whereby spatial relations can be assessed (**Fig. 1**). To evaluate feasibility and determine device size for LAAO, multiplanar axial, coronal, and sagittal reconstructions (MPR) are required to define and/or measure the LAA shape, orifice, landing zone, and depth. At the authors' institution, they use an oblique view of the LAA, which is obtained by tilting the axis in the sagittal and axial projections, representing a right anterior oblique 30° and cranial 10° projection in the coronal projection (**Fig. 7**). Hereby, the circumflex coronary artery, the upper left pulmonary vein ridge, and the LAA ostium are visualized in most cases (see **Fig. 7**, 3rd row and **Video 1**). As a consequence of the variable LAA anatomy, it may be necessary to prioritize the circumflex coronary artery or the pulmonary vein ridge rather than both. Because of the different design of devices, different definitions of the orifice and landing zone are used.[12,41]

Step-by-step approach to cardiac CT for LAAO		
(Using a Siemens Somatom Force 196-dual source scanner)		
Sublingual nitroglycerin 0.8 mg is administered to all patients.		

1. Topogram (overview of the chest)

2. Calcium score

3. Test bolus 10 mL contrast(350 mg I/mL concentration) followed by 50 mL saline. Flow rate 5.0 – 6.0 mL/s.

4. The scan delay is calculated in DynEva (Siemens). First ROI is placed in the left atrial appendage, second ROI in ascending aorta.

5. LAAO scan: first scan craniocaudal (first delay) followed by a caudocranial scan (second delay). To minimize the time between the 2 scans, no automatic breath hold is used. However, manual breath hold is essential.

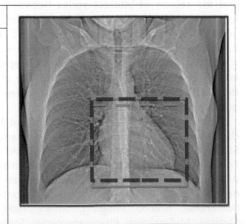

Fig. 6. Cardiac CT approach. ROI, region of interest.

Table 1
Aarhus University Hospital cardiac computed tomographic protocol for left atrial appendage occlusion using a 196 Dual-Source Scanner (Siemens SOMATOM Force)

	Sinus Rhythm	Arrhythmia/AF
Gating	Prospective ECG-gated	Prospective ECG-gated
Acquisition technique	High-pitch single-heart beat spiral	Double high-pitch single-heart beat spiral with 4-s delayed imaging
Scan direction	Craniocaudal	Craniocaudal followed by caudocranial
Tube potential	Primarily use automatic CarekV with optional manual correction: 40–80 kg: 70–80 kV 80–100 kg: 90–110 kV 100–130 kg: 120–130 kV >140 kg: 140–150 kV	
Tube current	Automated tube current modulation (CareDose)	
Slice thickness	0.70–0.75 mm	
Contrast medium	350 mg I/mL iodine concentration	
Contrast volume	40–60 mL adjusted to renal function and body weight	
Flow rate	5–6 mL/s	
Reconstruction phase	Heart rate <70 bpm: Diastolic phase (~65% R-R interval) Heart rate ≥70 bpm: Systolic phase (~40% R-R interval)	
Reconstructive kernel	Bv40 using iterative reconstruction (ADMIRE 3)	

Abbreviations: bpm, beats per minute; ECG, electrocardiogram.

The ACP and Amulet consist of a lobe and disc, whereby the disc is intended to cover the echocardiographic orifice, whereas the lobe is anchored 10 to 12 mm distally to the orifice.[52,53] Thus, 2 diameters must be determined for device sizing. A double-oblique projection is obtained by aligning the axis in the coronal and sagittal view through the plane of the echocardiographic orifice. Thereby, an "en face" view of the orifice is obtained in the axial projection (see **Fig. 7**, 4th row). The maximum and minimum diameters are measured. Similar measurements are obtained for the landing zone 10 to 12 mm inside the body of the LAA. Here, a plane perpendicular to the LAA wall is defined and the orthogonal axes are aligned to obtain a projection of the landing zone in the axial projection.

For the Watchman device, the dimensions of the anatomic orifice are used for selection of the device. The double-oblique en face view of the orifice is obtained after aligning the axis with the orifice plane in the sagittal and coronal view (**Fig. 8**, 3rd row). For the Watchman device, it is crucial to assess the depth of the LAA. Depth is measured from a central point of the orifice to the apex of the main lobe and should be as deep as the diameter of the chosen device. The depth may be obtained using MPR, but some investigators suggest using maximum intensity projections because of the angulations of the LAA.[38,41,46,54]

The appropriate device size is determined using the manufacturers' sizing guidelines. Device sizing is based on the maximum diameter, with a typical 3- to 5-mm upsizing for both devices.[20,52] The shape of the orifice or landing zone should be noted when sizing, especially if the shape is markedly elliptical. Oversizing should be more conservative in such cases. Some investigators have described promising outcomes using mean diameter, perimeter, or area-derived diameters.[39,40] This approach may be applicable, especially in the case of pronounced eccentricity. However, these results need further validation.

PREPROCEDURAL CARDIAC COMPUTED TOMOGRAPHY COMPARED WITH OTHER IMAGING MODALITIES

Few studies are available comparing cardiac CT, TEE, and angiography for LAAO. Most are retrospective, single-center studies, with small sample sizes. However, they consistently report larger dimensions found by cardiac CT than 2-dimensional (2D)/3D-TEE and angiography. Cardiac CT maximum diameter measurements are reported 2 to 5 mm larger than 2D-TEE measurements.[37–40,46] Similar results are found when cardiac CT is compared with 3D-TEE.[11,38,55] In an ACP series of 37 patients, cardiac CT and

Multiplanar reconstructed images, with the axial, sagittal and coronal views in 90-degree angles.

Axial view: Tilt axis 30-degree right anterior oblique.

Sagittal view: Tilt the axis 10-degree cranial.

Coronal view: The resulting RAO 30-degree and cranial 10-degree projection. Here, scroll in and out to obtain a view of the LAA, circumflex coronary artery and LUPV.

Orifice measurements

Coronal view: The crosshair is positioned at the orifice and the axial axis (yellow line) is aligned with the circumflex coronary artery andthe left upper pulmonary vein ridge.

The LAA depth can be measured.

Axial view: *En face* view of the orifice.

Maximum and minimum diameter can be measured.

Landing zone measurements

Coronal view: Sweep 10–12 mm inside the body of the LAA. The axial axis (yellow) should be perpendicular to the LAA neck.

Sagittal view: The axial axis (yellow line) is aligned perpendicular to the neck.

Axial view: The *en face* view of the landing zone.

Maximum and minimum diameters can be measured

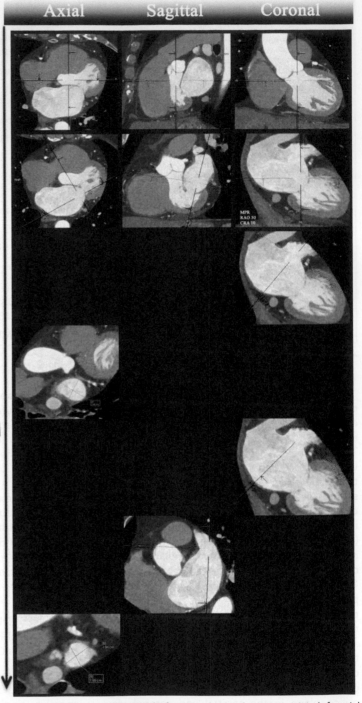

Fig. 7. Illustrated approach for analysis of preprocedural cardiac CT before Amulet implantation. LAA, left atrial appendage; LUPV, left upper pulmonary vein; RAO, right anterior oblique.

2D-TEE agreed on device size in 45.9% of cases.[56] A series of 73 Watchman implantations found that 2D-TEE and cardiac CT maximum diameter only agreed on device size in 25.4%.[39] A high eccentricity of the orifice increases the discrepancy between TEE and CT.[39] Clemente and colleagues[40] reported that peridevice leaks were more frequent with devices smaller than predicted by preprocedural CT. In a prospective study using cardiac CT,

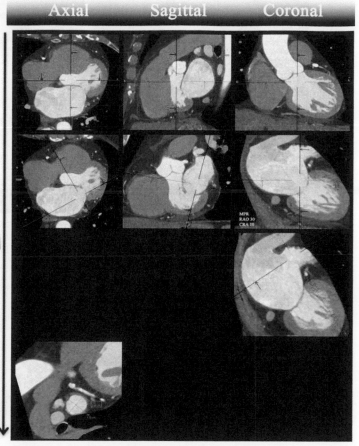

Multiplanar reconstructed images, with the axial, sagittal and coronal views in 90-degree angles.

Axial view: Tilt axis 30-degree right anterior oblique.

Sagittal view: Tilt the axis 10-degree cranial.

Coronal view: The resulting RAO 30-degree and cranial 10-degree projection. Here, scroll in and out to obtain a view of the LAA, circumflex coronary artery and LUPV.

Orifice measurements

Coronal view: The crosshair is positioned at the anatomical orifice and the axial axis (yellow line) is aligned with the circumflex coronary artery and a point 1–2 cm inside the left upper pulmonary vein ridge.

2D diameter and depth can be measured in this view.

Axial view: The maximum and minimum diameter of the orifice can be measured in the corresponding axial *en face* view

Fig. 8. Illustrated approach for analysis of preprocedural cardiac CT before Watchman implantation. LAA, left atrial appendage; LUPV, left upper pulmonary vein; RAO, right anterior oblique.

supplemented by 3D-printed models in the case of ambiguous anatomy, 19% of patients would incorrectly have been excluded based on 2D-TEE measurements of LAA length.[38] In turn, 3D-TEE would have undersized the device in 52.8% of cases. Thus, data support that cardiac CT provides the largest measurements of the LAA orifice, landing zone, and depth, which might be explained by the superior imaging quality of cardiac CT. The clinical impact hereof appears promising[38]; however, further studies are warranted.

POSTPROCEDURAL DEVICE-SURVEILLANCE WITH CARDIAC COMPUTED TOMOGRAPHY

Device surveillance after LAAO should include evaluation of peridevice leakage, device-related thrombosis, device positioning, and relation to surrounding cardiac structures. Traditionally, TEE has been used for evaluation, and especially, to define and evaluate peridevice

leaks in most clinical studies.[2–5,57] Cardiac CT cannot quantify peridevice flow, but residual peridevice leakage is reported in terms of peridevice gaps and contrast filling/opacification in the LAA (**Fig. 9**). A completely occluded LAA is most often defined as no visual peridevice gaps, and contrast attenuation less than 100 HU distally to the device, with less than 25% contrast opacification compared with the left atrium.[45,58] A standardized approach for obtainment of the standard projections of post-LAAO cardiac CT scans has been described by Behnes and colleagues.[43] The approach resembles the principles used for preprocedural planning of the LAAO.

The available data indicate that cardiac CT may be a more sensitive modality than TEE to detect peridevice leakage. Saw and colleagues[45] reported follow-up with cardiac CT in 44 patients, whereby contrast filling was found in 63.6% on cardiac CT, whereas only 13.6% had a peridevice leak detected on TEE at end of the LAAO procedure. Both CT and TEE were

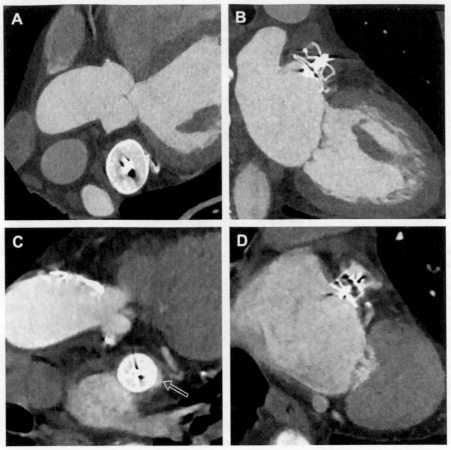

Fig. 9. Follow-up cardiac CT. (*A, B*) Completely sealed LAA, with no peridevice gaps (*A*) or contrast opacification distal to the device (*B*). (*C, D*) A well-positioned Amulet device, with a small peridevice gap (*C, arrow*), and contrast opacification distal to the lobe (*D*).

performed in 23 patients at follow-up, and contrast leakage was present in 12 (52%) on CT, whereas peridevice leak was present in 8 (35%) on TEE. Jaguszewski and colleagues[42] performed TEE and cardiac CT follow-up in 24 patients after ACP implantation and reported similar results; cardiac CT detected leaks in 62%, whereas TEE found only 36%. The reported average leak size with CT was 1.5 ± 1.4 mm, and 1.1 ± 1.6 mm with TEE. Lim and colleagues[58] reported that of 23 patients with no leak on TEE, 12 (52%) had a leak detected by cardiac CT. Cardiac CT may offer a superior sensitivity for leakage detection; however, the clinical significance of residual leaks remains unclear.[59]

Cardiac CT may readily assess device position and appears to be superior to TEE for determining off-axis device positions.[45] A perpendicular axis of the lobe in relation to the LAA neck appears critical to avoid residual leakage, and device compression greater than 10% seems to be associated with complete sealing.[40,42,45]

ADVANTAGES OF CARDIAC COMPUTED TOMOGRAPHY

The high spatial resolution of cardiac CT is a key advantage. It allows comprehensive visualization of the heart both preprocedurally and postprocedurally. The reproducibility is high,[55] and the acquisition allows for repeated manipulation of images. In turn, the scan is performed with patients being in a euvolemic state, which seems to be crucial because both size and volume of the LAA change with volume status.[60,61] This could be part of the explanation why measurements obtained by cardiac CT appear consistently larger than TEE.

The available data suggest a potential benefit in predicting device size; however, the results needs validation in a controlled, randomized setting.[38,40,56] The operator gains valuable anatomic information from preprocedural cardiac CT, which allows prediction of potential challenges during the procedure. In a postprocedural setting, the current data on cardiac CT are very limited, but indicate a superior sensitivity to detect leaks and evaluate device positioning.[42,45]

From a patient perspective, the noninvasive nature, fast acquisition, and nonfasting requirements limit the discomfort. The need for a less invasive alternative to TEE is supported by reports of 10% to 20% of patients refusing or unwilling to undergo TEE examination during the follow-up after LAAO.[42,62] In these cases, cardiac CT may be an alternative.

LIMITATIONS

The associated radiation exposure and subsequent risk should be acknowledged. The true quantification of radiation-induced cancer risk seems difficult,[63,64] and, moreover, improvements in scanner technology including dose reducing strategies have rapidly reduced the radiation associated with cardiac CT over the past decade.

The risk of contrast-induced nephropathy is a limitation; however, the incidence of contrast-induced acute kidney injury is less than 1% in standard patients undergoing elective contrast-enhanced imaging. The incidence is reported to be 4% in patients with chronic kidney disease.[65–68]

SUMMARY

Cardiac CT offers superior spatial resolution and imaging of the LAA and is a feasible alternative to TEE for guiding of LAAO. The available data indicate that cardiac CT may be better at predicting device size to determine feasibility of LAAO. Similarly, cardiac CT appears to have superior sensitivity for detection of residual leaks and evaluation of device positioning in the follow-up phase after LAAO. However, further studies are warranted.

SUPPLEMENTARY DATA

Supplementary data related to this article can be found online at https://doi.org/10.1016/j.iccl. 2017.12.004.

REFERENCES

1. Blackshear JL, Odell JA. Appendage obliteration to reduce stroke in cardiac surgical patients with atrial fibrillation. Ann Thorac Surg 1996;61(2):755–9.
2. Reddy VY, Sievert H, Halperin J, et al. Percutaneous left atrial appendage closure vs warfarin for atrial fibrillation: a randomized clinical trial. JAMA 2014; 312(19):1988–98.
3. Holmes DR, Kar S, Price MJ, et al. Prospective randomized evaluation of the Watchman left atrial appendage closure device in patients with atrial fibrillation versus long-term warfarin therapy: the PREVAIL trial. J Am Coll Cardiol 2014;64(1):1–12.
4. Tzikas A, Shakir S, Gafoor S, et al. Left atrial appendage occlusion for stroke prevention in atrial fibrillation: multicentre experience with the AMPLATZER cardiac plug. EuroIntervention 2016; 11(10):1170–9.
5. Landmesser U, Schmidt B, Nielsen-Kudsk JE, et al. Left atrial appendage occlusion with the AMPLATZER Amulet device: periprocedural and early clinical/echocardiographic data from a global prospective observational study. EuroIntervention 2017. https://doi.org/10.4244/EIJ-D-17-00493.
6. Boersma LV, Ince H, Kische S, et al. Efficacy and safety of left atrial appendage closure with WATCHMAN in patients with or without contraindication to oral anticoagulation: 1-year follow-up outcome data of the EWOLUTION trial. Heart Rhythm 2017. https://doi.org/10.1016/j.hrthm.2017. 05.038.
7. Boersma LVA, Schmidt B, Betts TR, et al. Implant success and safety of left atrial appendage closure with the WATCHMAN device: peri-procedural outcomes from the EWOLUTION registry. Eur Heart J 2016;37(31):2465–74.
8. Kirchhof P, Benussi S, Kotecha D, et al. 2016 ESC guidelines for the management of atrial fibrillation developed in collaboration with EACTS: the Task Force for the management of atrial fibrillation of the European Society of Cardiology (ESC) developed with the special contribution of the European Heart Rhythm Association (EHRA) of the ESC endorsed by the European Stroke Organisation (ESO). Eur Heart J 2016;37(38):2893–962.
9. Meier B, Blaauw Y, Khattab AA, et al. EHRA/EAPCI expert consensus statement on catheter-based left atrial appendage occlusion. EuroIntervention 2015; 10(9):1109–25.
10. Cabrera JA, Saremi F, Sánchez-Quintana D. Left atrial appendage: anatomy and imaging landmarks pertinent to percutaneous transcatheter occlusion. Heart 2014;100(20):1636–50.
11. Nucifora G, Faletra FF, Regoli F, et al. Evaluation of the left atrial appendage with real-time 3-dimensional transesophageal echocardiography: Implications for catheter-based left atrial appendage closure. Circ Cardiovasc Imaging 2011;4(5):514–23.
12. Veinot JP, Harrity PJ, Gentile F, et al. Anatomy of the normal left atrial appendage: a quantitative study of age-related changes in 500 autopsy hearts: implications for echocardiographic examination. Circulation 1997;96(9):3112–5.

13. Beigel R, Wunderlich NC, Ho SY, et al. The left atrial appendage: anatomy, function, and noninvasive evaluation. JACC Cardiovasc Imaging 2014;7(12):1251–65.

14. Wang Y, Di Biase L, Horton RP, et al. Left atrial appendage studied by computed tomography to help planning for appendage closure device placement. J Cardiovasc Electrophysiol 2010;21(9):973–82.

15. Halkin A, Cohen C, Rosso R, et al. Left atrial appendage and pulmonary artery anatomic relationship by cardiac-gated computed tomography: Implications for late pulmonary artery perforation by left atrial appendage closure devices. Heart Rhythm 2016;13(10):2064–9.

16. Di Biase L, Santangeli P, Anselmino M, et al. Does the left atrial appendage morphology correlate with the risk of stroke in patients with atrial fibrillation? Results from a multicenter study. J Am Coll Cardiol 2012;60(6):531–8.

17. Lupercio F, Carlos Ruiz J, Briceno DF, et al. Left atrial appendage morphology assessment for risk stratification of embolic stroke in patients with atrial fibrillation: a meta-analysis. Heart Rhythm 2016;13(7):1402–9.

18. Murarka S, Lazkani M, Moualla S, et al. Left atrial anatomy and patient-related factors associated with adverse outcomes with the Watchman device—a real world experience. J Interv Cardiol 2017;30(2):163–9.

19. Freixa X, Tzikas A, Basmadjian A, et al. The chicken-wing morphology: an anatomical challenge for left atrial appendage occlusion. J Interv Cardiol 2013;26(5):509–14.

20. Saw J, Lempereur M. Percutaneous left atrial appendage closure: procedural techniques and outcomes. JACC Cardiovasc Interv 2014;7(11):1205–20.

21. Romero J, Cao JJ, Garcia MJ, et al. Cardiac imaging for assessment of left atrial appendage stasis and thrombosis. Nat Rev Cardiol 2014;11(8):470–80.

22. Dorenkamp M, Sohns C, Vollmann D, et al. Detection of left atrial thrombus during routine diagnostic work-up prior to pulmonary vein isolation for atrial fibrillation: role of transesophageal echocardiography and multidetector computed tomography. Int J Cardiol 2013;163(1):26–33.

23. Kim YY, Klein AL, Halliburton SS, et al. Left atrial appendage filling defects identified by multidetector computed tomography in patients undergoing radiofrequency pulmonary vein antral isolation: a comparison with transesophageal echocardiography. Am Heart J 2007;154(6):1199–205.

24. Feuchtner GM, Dichtl W, Bonatti JO, et al. Diagnostic accuracy of cardiac 64-slice computed tomography in detecting atrial thrombi. Comparative study with transesophageal echocardiography and cardiac surgery. Invest Radiol 2008;43(11):794–801.

25. Hur J, Kim YJ, Lee H-J, et al. Left atrial appendage thrombi in stroke patients: detection with two-phase cardiac CT angiography versus transesophageal echocardiography. Radiology 2009;251(3):683–90.

26. Hur J, Pak H-N, Kim YJ, et al. Dual-enhancement cardiac computed tomography for assessing left atrial thrombus and pulmonary veins before radiofrequency catheter ablation for atrial fibrillation. Am J Cardiol 2013;112(2):238–44.

27. Hur J, Kim YJ, Lee H-J, et al. Dual-enhanced cardiac CT for detection of left atrial appendage thrombus in patients with stroke: a prospective comparison study with transesophageal echocardiography. Stroke 2011;42(9):2471–7.

28. Romero J, Husain SA, Kelesidis I, et al. Detection of left atrial appendage thrombus by cardiac computed tomography in patients with atrial fibrillation. Circ Cardiovasc Imaging 2013;6(2):185–94.

29. Zou H, Zhang Y, Tong J, et al. Multidetector computed tomography for detecting left atrial/left atrial appendage thrombus: a meta-analysis. Intern Med J 2015;45(10):1044–53.

30. Lazoura O, Ismail TF, Pavitt C, et al. A low-dose, dual-phase cardiovascular CT protocol to assess left atrial appendage anatomy and exclude thrombus prior to left atrial intervention. Int J Cardiovasc Imaging 2016;32(2):347–54.

31. Teunissen C, Habets J, Velthuis BK, et al. Double-contrast, single-phase computed tomography angiography for ruling out left atrial appendage thrombus prior to atrial fibrillation ablation. Int J Cardiovasc Imaging 2017;33(1):121–8.

32. Homsi R, Nath B, Luetkens JA, et al. Can contrast-enhanced multi-detector computed tomography replace transesophageal echocardiography for the detection of thrombogenic milieu and thrombi in the left atrial appendage: a prospective study with 124 patients. Rofo 2016;188(1):45–52.

33. Patel A, Au E, Donegan K, et al. Multidetector row computed tomography for identification of left atrial appendage filling defects in patients undergoing pulmonary vein isolation for treatment of atrial fibrillation: comparison with transesophageal echocardiography. Heart Rhythm 2008;5(2):253–60.

34. Hur J, Kim YJ, Lee H-J, et al. Cardioembolic stroke: dual-energy cardiac CT for differentiation of left atrial appendage thrombus and circulatory stasis. Radiology 2012;263(3):688–95.

35. Shapiro MD, Neilan TG, Jassal DS, et al. Multidetector computed tomography for the detection of

left atrial appendage thrombus. J Comput Assist Tomogr 2007;31(6):905–9.

36. Ismail TF, Panikker S, Markides V, et al. CT imaging for left atrial appendage closure: a review and pictorial essay. J Cardiovasc Comput Tomogr 2015;9(2):89–102.

37. Goitein O, Fink N, Hay I, et al. Cardiac CT Angiography (CCTA) predicts left atrial appendage occluder device size and procedure outcome. Int J Cardiovasc Imaging 2017;33(5):739–47.

38. Wang DD, Eng M, Kupsky D, et al. Application of 3-dimensional computed tomographic image guidance to WATCHMAN implantation and impact on early operator learning curve: single-center experience. JACC Cardiovasc Interv 2016; 9(22):2329–40.

39. Rajwani A, Nelson AJ, Shirazi MG, et al. CT sizing for left atrial appendage closure is associated with favourable outcomes for procedural safety. Eur Heart J Cardiovasc Imaging 2016. https://doi. org/10.1093/ehjci/jew212.

40. Clemente A, Avogliero F, Berti S, et al. Multimodality imaging in preoperative assessment of left atrial appendage transcatheter occlusion with the Amplatzer cardiac plug. Eur Heart J Cardiovasc Imaging 2015;16(11):1276–87.

41. Saw J, Lopes JP, Reisman M, et al. Cardiac computed tomography angiography for left atrial appendage closure. Can J Cardiol 2016;32(8): 1033.e1–9.

42. Jaguszewski M, Manes C, Puippe G, et al. Cardiac CT and echocardiographic evaluation of peri-device flow after percutaneous left atrial appendage closure using the AMPLATZER cardiac plug device. Catheter Cardiovasc Interv 2014;85(2):306–12.

43. Behnes M, Akin I, Sartorius B, et al. –LAA Occluder View for post-implantation Evaluation (LOVE)–standardized imaging proposal evaluating implanted left atrial appendage occlusion devices by cardiac computed tomography. BMC Med Imaging 2016; 16(1):25.

44. Kwong Y, Troupis J. Cardiac CT imaging in the context of left atrial appendage occlusion. J Cardiovasc Comput Tomogr 2015;9(1):13–8.

45. Saw J, Fahmy P, DeJong P, et al. Cardiac CT angiography for device surveillance after endovascular left atrial appendage closure. Eur Heart J Cardiovasc Imaging 2015;16(11):1198–206.

46. Saw J, Fahmy P, Spencer R, et al. Comparing measurements of CT angiography, TEE, and fluoroscopy of the left atrial appendage for percutaneous closure. J Cardiovasc Electrophysiol 2016; 27(4):414–22.

47. Sabarudin A, Sun Z, Ng K-H. A systematic review of radiation dose associated with different generations of multidetector CT coronary angiography. J Med Imaging Radiat Oncol 2012;56(1):5–17.

48. Sabarudin A, Sun Z. Coronary CT angiography: dose reduction strategies. World J Cardiol 2013; 5(12):465–72.

49. Mayo JR, Leipsic JA. Radiation dose in cardiac CT. AJR Am J Roentgenol 2009;192(3):646–53.

50. de Araújo Gonçalves P, Jerónimo Sousa P, Calé R, et al. Effective radiation dose of three diagnostic tests in cardiology: single photon emission computed tomography, invasive coronary angiography and cardiac computed tomography angiography. Rev Port Cardiol 2013;32(12):981–6.

51. Picano E, Vañó E, Rehani MM, et al. The appropriate and justified use of medical radiation in cardiovascular imaging: a position document of the ESC Associations of Cardiovascular Imaging, percutaneous cardiovascular interventions and electrophysiology. Eur Heart J 2014;35(10):665–72.

52. Tzikas A, Gafoor S, Meerkin D, et al. Left atrial appendage occlusion with the AMPLATZER Amulet device: an expert consensus step-by-step approach. EuroIntervention 2016;11(13):1512–21.

53. Park J-W, Bethencourt A, Sievert H, et al. Left atrial appendage closure with Amplatzer cardiac plug in atrial fibrillation: initial European experience. Catheter Cardiovasc Interv 2011;77(5):700–6.

54. Prakash R, Saw J. Imaging for percutaneous left atrial appendage closure. Catheter Cardiovasc Interv 2016;374:534.

55. Bai W, Chen Z, Tang H, et al. Assessment of the left atrial appendage structure and morphology: comparison of real-time three-dimensional transesophageal echocardiography and computed tomography. Int J Cardiovasc Imaging 2016. https://doi.org/10.1007/s10554-016-1044-4.

56. López Mínguez JR, González-Fernández R, Fernández-Vegas C, et al. Comparison of imaging techniques to assess appendage anatomy and measurements for left atrial appendage closure device selection. J Invasive Cardiol 2014;26(9):462–7.

57. Fountain RB, Holmes DR, Chandrasekaran K, et al. The PROTECT AF (WATCHMAN left atrial appendage system for embolic PROTECTion in patients with atrial fibrillation) trial. Am Heart J 2006; 151(5):956–61.

58. Lim Y-M, Kim J-S, Kim TH, et al. Delayed left atrial appendage contrast filling in computed tomograms after percutaneous left atrial appendage occlusion. J Cardiol 2017. https://doi.org/10.1016/j.jjcc.2017.04.007.

59. Viles Gonzalez JF, Kar S, Douglas P, et al. The clinical impact of incomplete left atrial appendage closure with the watchman device in patients with atrial fibrillation: a PROTECT AF (Percutaneous closure of the left atrial appendage versus warfarin therapy for prevention of stroke in patients with atrial fibrillation) substudy. J Am Coll Cardiol 2012;59(10):923–9.

60. Spencer RJ, DeJong P, Fahmy P, et al. Changes in left atrial appendage dimensions following volume loading during percutaneous left atrial appendage closure. JACC Cardiovasc Interv 2015;8(15):1935–41.

61. Al-Kassou B, Tzikas A, Stock F, et al. A comparison of two-dimensional and real-time 3D transoesophageal echocardiography and angiography for assessing the left atrial appendage anatomy for sizing a left atrial appendage occlusion system: impact of volume loading. EuroIntervention 2017; 12(17):2083–91.

62. Korsholm K, Nielsen KM, Jensen JM, et al. Transcatheter left atrial appendage occlusion in patients with atrial fibrillation and a high bleeding risk using aspirin alone for post-implant antithrombotic therapy. EuroIntervention 2016;12(17):2075–82.

63. Brenner DJ. What we know and what we don't know about cancer risks associated with radiation doses from radiological imaging. Br J Radiol 2014;87(1035):20130629.

64. Linet MS, Slovis TL, Miller DL, et al. Cancer risks associated with external radiation from diagnostic imaging procedures. CA Cancer J Clin 2012;62(2): 75–100.

65. Luk L, Steinman J, Newhouse JH. Intravenous contrast-induced nephropathy-the rise and fall of a threatening idea. Adv Chronic Kidney Dis 2017; 24(3):169–75.

66. Fukushima Y, Miyazawa H, Nakamura J, et al. Contrast-induced nephropathy (CIN) of patients with renal dysfunction in CT examination. Jpn J Radiol 2017;35(8):427–31.

67. Ozkok S, Ozkok A. Contrast-induced acute kidney injury: a review of practical points. World J Nephrol 2017;6(3):86–99.

68. Mamoulakis C, Tsarouhas K, Fragkiadoulaki I, et al. Contrast-induced nephropathy: basic concepts, pathophysiological implications and prevention strategies. Pharmacol Ther 2017. https://doi.org/ 10.1016/j.pharmthera.2017.06.009.

Incidence, Prevention, and Management of Periprocedural Complications of Left Atrial Appendage Occlusion

Jay Thakkar, MBBS, MD[a,b,c], Dimitra Vasdeki, MD[d],
Apostolos Tzikas, MD, PhD[d], Bernhard Meier, MD[e],
Jacqueline Saw, MD[f,*]

KEYWORDS

- Left atrial appendage occlusion • Device embolization • Periprocedural complications
- Pericardial effusion

KEY POINTS

- Major procedural complications related to left atrial appendage occlusion (LAAO) are relatively infrequent in contemporary practice (<1%–2%) but may be associated with major morbidity and mortality.
- LAAO operators should be knowledgeable about these potential complications and management.
- Often, prompt recognition and treatment are necessary to avoid rapid deterioration and dire consequences.
- With stringent guidelines on operator training and competency requirements, and on procedural-technical refinements, LAAO can be performed safely with low complications rates.
- LAAO is a feasible, safe, and effective alternative to oral anticoagulation for nonvalvular atrial fibrillation stroke prevention.

INTRODUCTION

The left atrial appendage (LAA) is a multilobed, embryologic remnant of the left atrium (LA) that exhibits highly variable and complex anatomy unique to each patient. Thus, LAA occlusion (LAAO) requires careful evaluation and planning on a case-by-case basis. Currently, the percutaneous endovascular approach is most widely used for LAAO. This technique requires transseptal puncture (TSP), which increases the risk of the procedure. The thin wall of the LAA and

Disclosure Statement: Within the past 12 months, the authors and their families have had a financial interest or arrangement or affiliation with these organizations. None (J. Thakkar and D. Vasdeki). Unrestricted research grant supports (from the Canadian Institutes of Health Research, Heart and Stroke Foundation of Canada, University of British Columbia Division of Cardiology, AstraZeneca, Abbott Vascular, St Jude Medical, Boston Scientific, and Servier); speaker honoraria (AstraZeneca, St Jude Medical, Boston Scientific, and Sunovion); consultancy and advisory board honoraria (AstraZeneca, St Jude Medical, and Abbott Vascular); and proctorship honoraria (St Jude Medical and Boston Scientific) (J. Saw). Speaker bureau Abbott (B. Meier). Dr A. Tzikas is a consultant and proctor for AbbottVascular.
[a] Vancouver General Hospital, University of British Columbia, Vancouver, British Columbia, Canada; [b] The George Institute for Global Health, Missenden Road, Camperdown, NSW 2050, Australia; [c] The University of Sydney, Broadway, NSW 2006, Australia; [d] AHEPA University Hospital, St. Kiriakidi 1, Thessaloniki 54637, Greece; [e] Department of Cardiology, University Hospital of Bern, Bern CH-3010, Switzerland; [f] Interventional Cardiology, Interventional Cardiology Fellowship Training Program, Vancouver General Hospital, University of British Columbia, 2775 Laurel Street, Level 9, Vancouver, British Columbia V5Z1M9, Canada
* Corresponding author.
E-mail address: jsaw@mail.ubc.ca

Intervent Cardiol Clin 7 (2018) 243–252
https://doi.org/10.1016/j.iccl.2017.12.008
2211-7458/18/© 2017 Elsevier Inc. All rights reserved.

manipulation of large-bore sheaths to achieve co-axial device delivery can increase the risk of perforation. The low flow-low pressure circulation of the LA also predisposes to thromboembolism and air embolism. Over the last decade, improved experience and meticulous technique has brought dramatic reduction in the incidence of major procedural complications (death, stroke, cardiac tamponade, device embolization).[1] Currently, the Watchman (Boston Scientific, Nattick, MA) and Amplatzer Cardiac Plug (ACP) or Amulet (Abbott Vascular Inc, Minneapolis, MN) are most commonly implanted worldwide; hence this article mainly focuses on these devices. Table 1 provides a summary of the major complications reported across leading trials of LAAO.

PERICARDIAL EFFUSION AND CARDIAC TAMPONADE
Incidence
Pericardial effusion is the most common complication after LAAO. The incidence of pericardial effusion has declined over time with improved operator skills. In the Percutaneous Closure of

the Left Atrial Appendage Versus Warfarin Therapy for Prevention of Stroke in Patients with Atrial Fibrillation (PROTECT AF) trial, 2009, the first landmark LAA closure study using the Watchman device, pericardial effusion requiring intervention was reported in 4.3% of the study population.[3] This has steadily declined since, with PREVAIL (Prospective Randomized Evaluation of the WATCHMAN LAA Closure Device in Patients with Atrial Fibrillation versus Long Term Warfarin Therapy), 2014, and the Continued Access Protocol Registry (CAP2) reporting a frequency of 1.9%.[1] The overall incidence of cardiac tamponade is approximately 1.3% in a pooled analysis of Watchman clinical trials and registries.[1] The frequency of pericardial effusion in early clinical trials with the ACP device ranged between 1.9% and 3.7%.[7,8] In the most recently published Amulet Postmarketing Registry of 1088 patients, the incidence of cardiac tamponade was 1.2%.[9]

Classification
The Munich LAA consensus document classified pericardial effusion based on timing of occurrence

Table 1
Procedure-related complications reported across major left atrial appendage occlusion trials and registries

Study	Study Features	Pericardial Tamponade (%) or Surgical Treatment (%)	Stroke (%)	Device Embolism (%)	Mortality (%)	Vascular or Major Bleeding (%)
Holmes et al,[2] 2009 PROTECT AF	Watchman RCT N = 707 I = 463	22 (4.8) or 7 (1.5)	5 (1.1)	3 (0.6)	0 (0)	1 (0.2) or 16 (3.5)[a]
Holmes et al,[4] 2014 PREVAIL	Watchman RCT N = 407 I = 269	5 (1.9) or 1 (0.4)	1 (0.4)	2 (0.7)	0 (0)	1 (0.4) or 1 (0.4)[b]
Reddy et al,[3] 2011 CAP	Watchman registry N = 460	8 (1.4) or 1 (0.2)	0 (0)	1 (0.2)	0 (0)	1(0.2) or 3 (0.7)[c]
CAP2						
Boersma et al,[5] 2016 EWOLUTION	Watchman registry N = 1019	2 (0.2) or NA	1 (0.1)	2 (0.2)	1 (0.1)	4 (0.4) or 7 (0.7)[d]
Tzikas et al,[6] 2016	ACP retrospective analysis multicenter N = 1047	13 (1.24) or NA	9 (0.9)	8 (0.8)	8 (0.76)	4 (0.4) or 13 (1.24)[e]

Abbreviations: CAP, continued access protocol; I, intervention (device) group subjects; N, total enrolled subjects; NA, not available; RCT, randomized controlled trial.
  [a] Arteriovenous fistula in 1 subject and major bleeding defined as greater than 2 units of packed red blood cells or surgical intervention in 16 subjects.
  [b] Arteriovenous fistula in 1 subject and major bleeding in 1 subject.
  [c] Pseudoaneurysm in 1 subject and bleeding in 3 subjects.
  [d] Vascular damage to the groin in 4 subjects and major bleeding per Bleeding Academic Research Consortium criteria.
  [e] Pseudoaneurysm in 3 subjects and arteriovenous fistula in 1 subject, 8 subjects had bleeding from femoral artery and its association with the LAA procedure was not clear, 1 subject had pulmonary artery perforation, and 2 subjects had gastrointestinal bleeding.

and severity based on interventional treatment required.[10] Pericardial effusion was categorized as intraprocedural, acute ($\leq$48 hours from the index procedure), or late (>48 hours from the index procedure). An effusion requiring percutaneous or surgical drainage, or blood transfusion, or resulting in shock or death, was considered clinically relevant (significant). For procedures using the epicardial approach for LAAO, clinically relevant effusion was defined as aspiration of greater than 500 mL of bloody fluid, need for blood transfusion, or surgical intervention.

Mechanism

Most pericardial effusions occur early, 89% within 24 hours of the procedure, and are due to procedural mishaps.[3] Manipulation of the guidewires, catheters, device delivery sheaths, and transseptal needles can be associated with trauma to the LAA, LA, or pulmonary veins. The hooks on these endovascular LAA devices may also penetrate the thin LAA wall, with accentuated risk during recapturing or repositioning of the devices. However, in approximately 30% of cases, the cause of pericardial effusion could not be identified.[3] With the LARIAT (SentreHeart, Redwood City, CA) or other epicardial devices, the dry pericardial tap required can inadvertently penetrate cardiac chambers.

Prevention

- Obtain a baseline assessment of the pericardial space; for example, with a transesophageal echocardiogram (TEE). This is important to exclude preexisting chronic effusion, which is not uncommon.
- If feasible, oral anticoagulation (OAC) should be interrupted before LAAO. Patients at high risk for stroke off anticoagulation may continue anticoagulation through the day of procedure, or bridging therapy may be considered.
- Procedural guidance with TEE or intracardiac echocardiography (ICE) should be used for safe TSP. Tenting of the septum with the needle must be visualized before puncturing the septum (typically in 2 views: long and short axis on TEE). Tenting can also be documented by fluoroscopy with dye injection. Transmitted pulsation, when felt by the operator, implies close proximity to ascending aorta and the needle should be repositioned; clockwise rotation will direct the needle tip posteriorly. The risk of perforating the LA is higher when septum is thick or aneurysmal and leathery, in which case a radiofrequency needle or Bovie cautery

can be useful. Alternatively, the stylet of the TSP or the back-end of a coronary wire can be used to help the needle penetrate the stiff septum. Specialized needle-free systems, such as SafeSept (Pressure Products Inc, San Pedro, CA) are available for TSP.
- A pigtail catheter should be used to safely navigate the device delivery sheath into the LAA. Angiography of the LAA should be performed via the pigtail catheter or via the sheath after removing the dilator with hand (or low-volume power) injection.
- Because the LAA is a blind-ended structure, any wire should be advanced cautiously and only under fluoroscopic guidance. Note that even a soft J-wire can perforate the thinned-walled LAA when it is advanced out a catheter against the LAA wall.
- Early detection of a pericardial effusion is crucial. An invasive arterial pressure line (ie, radial) can allow for immediate recognition of hemodynamic compromise due to pericardial effusion. The TEE operator should check periodically for the presence of a new effusion. Unsedated patients will invariably indicate chest pain when blood enters the pericardium. In contrast to chest pain due to air embolism, there will be no electrocardiographic changes.
- When deep intubation of the LAA is needed, the device delivery sheath must be advanced over a pigtail catheter and tenting of the LAA wall by the sheath should be avoided.
- A pericardial drainage kit should be readily available in the catheterization laboratory.
- LAAO should be performed at a site with cardiac or, at least, thoracic surgical backup.

Treatment

- Early recognition, prompt hemodynamic resuscitation, and percutaneous drainage are fundamental. Intravascular volume expansion and administration of inotropes is often required while emergency pericardiocentesis is being performed.
- Emergency pericardiocentesis is commonly performed via subxiphoid approach. Parasternal or apical access may be easier in obese patients. Fluoroscopic guidance in anteroposterior and lateral views is helpful.

- The Micropuncture Access Set (Cook Medical, Bloomington, IN) may be used to minimize trauma while trying to access the pericardial space. A 21-gauge 7-cm long needle is used to advance a 40-cm long 0.018-inch wire under fluoroscopy. The needle is then exchanged for a 4F or 5F 10-cm long dilator-catheter assembly. The micropuncture dilator-wire is then withdrawn, allowing blood suctioning or pressure interrogation to confirm position in pericardial sac before advancing a stiffer 0.035-inch wire, followed by the wide bore pericardial drain.
- If the micropuncture kit needle is not long enough, it may be replaced with a long spinal needle. Spinal needles are still significantly smaller (18–21 gauge) in caliber than the usual needle provided in most conventional pericardiocentesis kits (18 gauge). After the needle and trocar of the spinal needle have been introduced beyond the skin, the trocar is removed and the needle advanced with aspiration on a syringe attached to the needle.
- An overt cardiac perforation with persistent active bleeding is rare (<0.5%) and typically requires surgical intervention. Autotransfusion must be considered to minimize blood loss and the need for transfusion. Timing of anticoagulation reversal is still a matter of debate. Early reversal can be associated with clotting in the pericardial space and blocking the pericardial drain. This may lead to refractory tamponade and hemodynamic collapse. Reversal of anticoagulation and administration of clotting factors should be deferred until pericardial drainage has been achieved, or when operative team is activated and emergency sternotomy is imminent.[11]
- Of note, if the delivery sheath has perforated into the pericardial sac, it should be left in position until pericardial drainage is achieved, and the surgical team is ready for emergency thoracotomy. It may be possible to insert a septal occluder across the pericardial perforation to seal the hole.[12]

DEVICE EMBOLIZATION
Incidence, Mechanisms, and Clinical Presentation
Device embolization remains one of the most feared complication of the LAAO procedure. Recent data from Watchman clinical trials and registries reported an average incidence of 0.25%.[1] One systematic review[13] of device embolization with Watchman (13 cases) and ACP (18 cases) examined the timing and location of embolized devices. Most device embolizations (69%) were acute but 31% were detected late (1–7 months) but were probably early embolizations that were missed. Solid adhesion to the wall can occur within days according to animal studies. This underscores the need for confirmation of correct position within 24 hours postprocedure. The embolized devices were located in the left ventricle (43%), aorta (43%), and LA (14%). It is generally thought that the final location of an embolized device is a function of device size. Larger devices are more likely to be trapped in the narrower left ventricular outflow tract. **Table 2** outlines potential mechanisms underlying device embolization. The clinical presentation after hospital discharge is a function of the location of embolized device. Most embolizations are clinically silent; however, palpitations, heart failure, hypotension, and cardiac arrest have been described in cases of obstructed cardiac outflow. A management algorithm is outlined in **Fig. 1**.

Prevention
- Detailed assessment of LAA size and axis will help select a suitable device type and size. For a very shallow LAA, a device with a shorter profile may be preferred.[14]
- Supplemental imaging using preprocedural cardiac computed tomography scan is a valuable tool to help plan the procedure.

Table 2 Mechanisms underlying left atrial appendage occlusion device embolization	
Device size	Implanted device is too small or generously oversized
Device position	Shallow implant (too proximal) or off-axis
Operator-related	Vigorous tug testing
Patient-related	Spontaneous reversion to sinus rhythm (restores LAA contractility) Vigorous physical movement before device is sufficiently adherent
Miscellaneous	Therapeutic cardioversion soon after device implantation

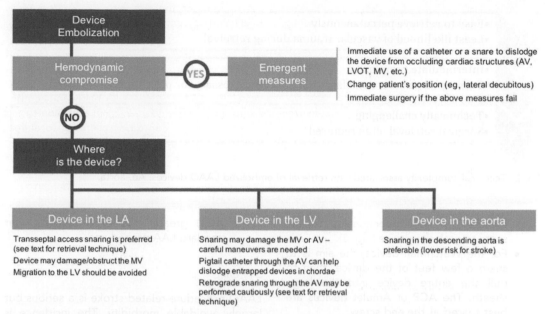

Fig. 1. Algorithm to manage device embolization. AV, aortic valve; LA, left atrium; LV, left ventricle; LVOT, left ventricular outflow tract; MV, mitral valve.

- Appropriate device oversizing is recommended (9%–25% for Watchman, 3–5 mm for ACP, and 2–4 mm for Amulet).
- Check the connection between the device and the delivery wire during device preparation to make sure device is connected.
- After device deployment, use the stability checkpoints and tests according to the manufacturers' instructions for use.
- Assess the device position in multiple views with 2-dimensional TEE and, ideally, with 3-dimensional TEE, or on fluoroscopy with dye injection using views without overlap of the LA and LAA, and of disc and lobe in case of Amplatzer occluders, before release.
- Delay a few minutes after device deployment in the LAA before releasing the cable, which will allow the device to expand and accommodate to its final position for self-expanding devices.
- Reassess the device position and signs of stability whenever a tug test is performed on angiography and TEE or ICE.
- Extra caution should be used for larger devices (>25 mm) because they may be lodged in the left ventricle in case of embolization, where it can be very challenging and risky to snare them.

- Most device embolizations occur early, thus surveillance TTE during the first 24 hours is highly recommended.

Percutaneous Retrieval of an Embolized Left Atrial Appendage Occlusion Device

- The choice of retrieval technique (**Fig. 2**) depends on the location of device and operator's experience.
- The percutaneous retrieval armamentarium should comprise large sheaths, loop-snares, and bioptomes.
- A larger sheath (≥2F–4F larger than the embolized device delivery sheath size) should be used; for example, 14F to 18F 80-cm length. Beveling the sheath tip increases the tip orifice, although care should be taken given the sharp edge to avoid perforation. In general, the gooseneck snares (120 cm) with a single large loop work much better than other types of snares (eg, Ensnare, with multiple loops). The size of gooseneck snare should generally be at least a 10-mm loop for ease of grabbing the device end screw or feet.
- The snare should be placed through a 5F to 6F coronary guiding catheter (eg, judkins right 4, extra backup) and, in turn, placed through the large retrieval sheath (the telescoping technique).[15] The guiding

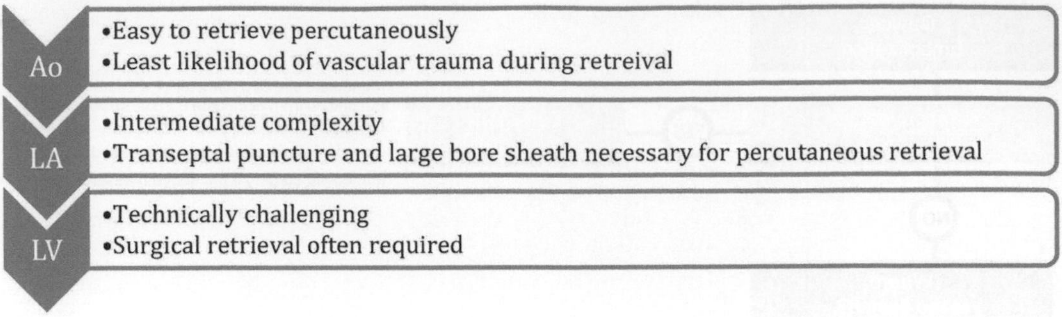

Ao	• Easy to retrieve percutaneously • Least likelihood of vascular trauma during retreival
LA	• Intermediate complexity • Transeptal puncture and large bore sheath necessary for percutaneous retrieval
LV	• Technically challenging • Surgical retrieval often required

Fig. 2. Technical complexity associated with retrieval of embolized LAAO devices. Ao, aorta.

catheter provides directionality to the snare to grab the device (Fig. 3).

- For the Watchman device, the aim is to snare a few feet of the device, then to pull the entire device into the large sheath. The ACP or Amulet devices are best snared at the end screw.
- The device must be pulled entirely within the sheath before removal of the sheath. If the device is partially stuck outside the retrieval sheath, a bioptome forceps may be used to pull the device in completely. As a last resort, the device and the still partially protruding device may be removed as a unit. In case of removal through an artery, preclosure with a suture should have been prepared or wire access must be preserved.
- Anticoagulation with heparin should be provided throughout the procedure, aiming for an activated clotting time

(ACT) greater than 250 seconds, per standard LAA procedures.

STROKE

LAAO procedure-related stroke is a serious but largely avoidable morbidity. The incidence is generally reported as less than 0.5%. This presents usually within 24 hours of the procedure. Most events are related to air embolism, occur immediately, and are reversible. Major mechanisms underlying stroke after LAAO are summarized in Table 3.

Air Embolism

Air embolism is a rare complication of LAAO and it is usually caused by poor technique. Air embolism to the cerebral circulation can cause a transient ischemic attack (TIA) or a stroke that may not be recognized if the patient is under general anesthesia. A clinical clue may be transient ST-segment elevation as a sign of simultaneous coronary air embolism. Air typically embolizes to the right coronary artery, which takes superiorly, and causes ST-segment elevation in inferior leads, hypotension, and/or bradycardia. In the PROTECT AF study, air embolism resulted in strokes in 1% (5 out of 463) of cases.[3] In a recent

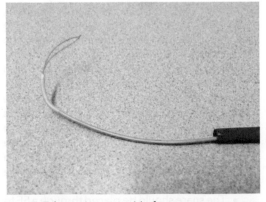

Fig. 3. Telescoping assembly for percutaneous snaring of embolized LAAO device. A 120 cm long Gooseneck snare is placed within a 100 cm long 5F to 6F coronary guide catheter, inside a 80 cm long 14F to 18F retrieval sheath.

Table 3
Mechanisms of stroke after left atrial appendage occlusion procedure

Early (Periprocedural)	Late (>7 d Postprocedure)
1. Air embolism 2. De novo thrombus formation on equipment 3. Embolism of preexisting LAA thrombus	1. Device-associated thrombus 2. Incomplete LAA closure 3. Non-LAA source of thrombus

series with refined procedural skills, severe air embolism were rare.

Prevention

- General anesthesia and endotracheal intubation with positive thoracic pressure can be protective of air embolism.
- Maintenance of left atrial pressure greater than 10 mm Hg (by administering saline) is another way to prevent air embolism and is recommended by most operators.
- A transseptal sheath may be used. After positioning the sheath in the LA, remove the wire and the dilator with a slow and steady motion, while keeping the proximal end (operator end) below the level of the heart. Always suction residual air from the connecting tubing and transducer before connecting and injecting the contrast.
- Meticulous flushing of all the catheters and careful device preparation as per instructions for use is mandatory.

Treatment

- The anatomy of the LAA, which is usually oriented superiorly, may result in air entrapment within it. Air can be aspirated by using a pigtail catheter. Device implantation may also be considered to trap the embolized air within the LAA, and the patient should remain supine for a few hours to prevent air dislodgement.
- Administration of 100% oxygen, the Trendelenburg position, and/or a hyperbaric chamber may be necessary, depending on the severity.

De Novo Equipment Associated with Thrombus Formation

Thrombus formation during LAAO can occur on the equipment or on the left atrial structures, potentially jeopardizing the procedure. Incomplete heparinization is the most common reason for thrombus formation, especially in cases of disruption of the endocardial surface. Another reason is the lack of flushing during longer intervals without manipulation; for example, during performing and assessment of echocardiographic pictures.

Management

- It is recommended to have an ACT greater than 250 seconds before introducing any equipment into the LA.

- In case of a difficult TSP, thrombus can develop on the TSP needle or sheath, thus, administering of heparin (eg, a half-dose) before TSP, followed by full heparinization after crossing the septum, may be desirable.
- The ACT should be periodically checked (every 20 minutes) and corrected.
- Thrombus is usually not visible on fluoroscopy, thus TEE surveillance is important for early detection.
- Depending on its position, size, and mobility, thrombus aspiration via a large sheath may be attempted.
- Thrombolysis with alteplase of equipment thrombosis may be attempted.
- If available, use of a cerebral protection device may be considered before starting any manipulations.

Embolism of a Preexisting Left Atrial Appendage Thrombus

Dislodgment of preexisting LAA thrombus not recognized at the time of the procedure can result in a disabling stroke. Thus, meticulous preprocedural TEE assessment for LAA thrombus is necessary. Often, dense swirls of spontaneous echo contrast (SEC) in the LAA can mimic a thrombus. The dynamically changing swirl patterns and marked reduction in echo-density after volume expansion (saline bolus to increase the mean LA pressure) may improve SEC, which may avoid unnecessary procedural deferment. Some operators prefer performing the procedure on OAC; however, if OAC is interrupted, bridging therapy with heparin should be considered in patients at very high stroke risk. Successful entrapment of preexisting thrombus in the LAA using ACP or Amulet devices has been described; however, this is not recommended routinely.[16]

DEVICE-RELATED COMPLICATIONS
Left Atrial Appendage Occlusion Device Associated with Thrombus

Device-associated thrombus (DAT) is usually clinically silent and detected on surveillance TEE at follow-up. In the PROTECT AF study, 20 subjects (4.2%) had DAT and 3 subjects had stroke (0.3% annualized stroke rate). A recent analysis from the prospective European EVOLUTION registry identified DAT in 2.6% and stroke in 0.4% of subjects.[17] The ACP multicenter study analyzed 344 follow-up TEEs in a core-laboratory, and identified DAT in 3.2% of subjects.[18] The ACP-associated thrombus had often been attached to the connector pin,[19] resulting in modification

Box 1
Mechanisms underlying peridevice leak
Noncircular LAA orifice shape (eg, oval, tear drop, irregular)
Device undersizing
Off-axis device deployment (malapposition against the LAA wall)
Postimplant device migration
Incomplete endothelialization
Remodeling of the LAA postimplant

of the second-generation Amulet device, which has a recessed proximal end screw. In a systematic review of 30 studies with 2118 implanted LAAO devices, DAT incidence was 3.9%, and approximately 7% of subjects had stroke or TIA.[20]

Management

- There is no consensus on screening for and management strategy for DAT.
- Surveillance imaging of the device postimplant should be performed at least once (45 days–6 months post-LAAO). Some operators advocate performing it twice (with additional late imaging at ~12 months).
- DAT should be treated if present because approximately 7% are associated with stroke or TIA.
- Treatment may consist of adding or intensifying anticoagulation for approximately 6 weeks.

- Anticoagulation may include OAC (warfarin or non-vitamin K–dependent oral anticoagulant), low-molecular-weight heparin, or intravenous heparin.
- Rarely, surgical thrombus excision may be required.

Peridevice Leaks

It has been proposed that inadequate sealing of the LAA cavity could be associated with persistent flow, thrombus formation, and embolic stroke. Mechanisms underlying persistent leaks after endovascular deployment are summarized in **Box 1**.

Management

- There is no consensus on a treatment threshold or definition of an acceptable peridevice leak. The threshold to define procedural success was less than 5 mm peridevice leak in the PROTECT AF and PREVAIL studies, whereas other studies or investigators used a more conservative threshold of less than 3 mm.
- Management may include continued OAC or implantation of a second LAAO device, which may include Amplatzer septal occluders, patent foramen ovale occluders, ACP or Amulet, or vascular or ductal occluders.[21]

OTHER COMPLICATIONS

Other complications that may occur during endovascular LAAO are summarized in **Table 4**.

Table 4		
Miscellaneous complications related to the left atrial appendage occlusion procedure		
Source	**Complications**	**Comments**
Access site	Bleeding Hematoma Pseudoaneurysm Infection Deep venous thrombosis	• Infrequent • Femoral vein puncture procedures are associated with lower complications compared with arterial punctures • Consider preclosure with Proglide (Abbott Vascular Inc, Minneapolis, MN) to secure hemostasis
TEE-related	Esophageal trauma	—
Anesthesia-related	Trauma to airway Aspiration pneumonia	• More common with general anesthesia
Technique-related	Pericarditis	• Common with devices requiring epicardial approach • Self-limiting • Requires non-steroidal anti-inflammatory drugs or colchicine
Other	Atrial arrhythmia	• Typically supraventricular tachycardia • Direct manipulation in atrium

SUMMARY

Major procedural complications related to LAAO are relatively infrequent in contemporary practice (<1%–2%) but may be associated with major morbidity and mortality. Therefore, LAAO operators should be knowledgeable about these potential complications and their management. Often, prompt recognition and treatment are necessary to avoid rapid deterioration and dire consequences. With stringent guidelines on operator training and competency requirements, and on procedural-technical refinements, LAAO can be performed safely with low complication rates. Thus, LAAO is a feasible, safe, and effective alternative to OAC for nonvalvular atrial fibrillation stroke prevention.

REFERENCES

1. Reddy VY, Gibson DN, Kar S, et al. Post-approval U.S. experience with left atrial appendage closure for stroke prevention in atrial fibrillation. J Am Coll Cardiol 2017;69(3):253–61.

2. Holmes DR, Reddy VY, Turi ZG, et al. Percutaneous closure of the left atrial appendage versus warfarin therapy for prevention of stroke in patients with atrial fibrillation: a randomised non-inferiority trial. Lancet 2009;374(9689):534–42.

3. Reddy VY, Holmes D, Doshi SK, et al. Safety of percutaneous left atrial appendage closure: results from the Watchman Left Atrial Appendage System for Embolic Protection in Patients with AF (PROTECT AF) clinical trial and the Continued Access Registry. Circulation 2011;123(4):417–24.

4. Holmes DR Jr, Kar S, Price MJ, et al. Prospective randomized evaluation of the Watchman Left Atrial Appendage Closure device in patients with atrial fibrillation versus long-term warfarin therapy: the PREVAIL trial. J Am Coll Cardiol 2014;64(1):1–12.

5. Boersma LV, Schmidt B, Betts TR, et al. Implant success and safety of left atrial appendage closure with the WATCHMAN device: peri-procedural outcomes from the EWOLUTION registry. Eur Heart J 2016;37(31):2465–74.

6. Tzikas A, Shakir S, Gafoor S, et al. Left atrial appendage occlusion for stroke prevention in atrial fibrillation: multicentre experience with the AMPLATZER Cardiac Plug. EuroIntervention 2016; 11(10):1170–9.

7. Park JW, Bethencourt A, Sievert H, et al. Left atrial appendage closure with Amplatzer cardiac plug in atrial fibrillation: initial European experience. Catheter Cardiovasc Interv 2011;77(5):700–6.

8. Urena M, Rodes-Cabau J, Freixa X, et al. Percutaneous left atrial appendage closure with the AMPLATZER cardiac plug device in patients with nonvalvular atrial fibrillation and contraindications to anticoagulation therapy. J Am Coll Cardiol 2013;62(2):96–102.

9. Landmesser U, Schmidt B, Nielsen-Kudsk JE, et al. Left atrial appendage occlusion with the AMPLATZER Amulet device: periprocedural and early clinical/echocardiographic data from a global prospective observational study. EuroIntervention 2017;13(7):867–76.

10. Tzikas A, Holmes JDR, Gafoor S, et al. Percutaneous left atrial appendage occlusion: the Munich consensus document on definitions, endpoints, and data collection requirements for clinical studies. Europace 2017;19(1):4–15.

11. Casserly IP, Walsh K, Saw J. Chapter 18-Procedural complications and management. In: Saw J, Kar S, Price MJ, editors. Left atrial appendage closure. Mechanical approaches to stroke prevention in atrial fibrillation. Switzerland: Humana Press, Springer International Publishing; 2016. p. 261–73.

12. Meier B, Tarbine SG, Costantini CR. Percutaneous management of left atrial appendage perforation during device closure. Catheter Cardiovasc Interv 2014;83(2):305–7.

13. Aminian A, Lalmand J, Tzikas A, et al. Embolization of left atrial appendage closure devices: a systematic review of cases reported with the watchman device and the amplatzer cardiac plug. Catheter Cardiovasc Interv 2015;86(1):128–35.

14. Saw J, Lempereur M. Percutaneous left atrial appendage closure: procedural techniques and outcomes. JACC Cardiovasc Interv 2014;7(11): 1205–20.

15. Fahmy P, Eng L, Saw J. Retrieval of embolized left atrial appendage devices. Catheter Cardiovasc Interv 2016. [Epub ahead of print].

16. Jalal Z, Iriart X, Dinet ML, et al. Extending percutaneous left atrial appendage closure indications using the AMPLATZER Cardiac Plug device in patients with persistent left atrial appendage thrombus: The thrombus trapping technique. Arch Cardiovasc Dis 2016;109(12):659–66.

17. Bergmann MW, Betts TR, Sievert H, et al. Early anticoagulation drug regimens after WATCHMAN left atrial appendage closure: safety and efficacy. EuroIntervention 2017;13(7):877–84.

18. Saw J, Tzikas A, Shakir S, et al. Incidence and Clinical Impact of Device-Associated Thrombus and Peri-Device Leak Following Left Atrial Appendage Closure With the Amplatzer Cardiac Plug. JACC Cardiovasc Interv 2017;10(4):391–9.

19. Fernandez-Rodriguez D, Vannini L, Martin-Yuste V, et al. Medical management of connector pin thrombosis with the Amplatzer cardiac plug left atrial closure device. World J Cardiol 2013;5(10):391–3.

20. Lempereur M, Aminian A, Freixa X, et al. Device-associated thrombus formation after left atrial

appendage occlusion: a systematic review of events reported with the Watchman, the Amplatzer Cardiac Plug and the Amulet. Catheter Cardiovasc Interv 2017. [Epub ahead of print].

21. Hornung M, Gafoor S, Id D, et al. Catheter-based closure of residual leaks after percutaneous occlusion of the left atrial appendage. Catheter Cardiovasc Interv 2016;87(7):1324–30.

Left Atrial Appendage Occlusion

The Current Device Landscape and Future Perspectives

Ignacio Cruz-Gonzalez, MD, PhD[a],*, Monica Fuertes-Barahona, MD[a], Jose C. Moreno-Samos, MD[a], Rocio Gonzalez-Ferreiro, MD[a], Yan Yin Lam, MD[b], Pedro L. Sanchez, MD, PhD[a]

KEYWORDS

- Atrial fibrillation • Stroke prevention • Left atrial appendage occlusion • Stroke

---

KEY POINTS

- Left atrial appendage occlusion is a safe and effective therapy for stroke prevention in atrial fibrillation patients.
- Different devices have been used for left atrial appendage occlusion.
- Several devices for left atrial appendage occlusion are under development or in the initial clinical experience.

Since the earliest designs of left atrial appendage occlusion (LAAO) devices, technological evolution has undergone a continuous advance resulting in significant improvements in the currently available devices.

In this article, the latest design improvements and clinical data regarding the most widely used devices, the Amplatzer Amulet (Abbott Vascular, Abbott Park, IL, USA) and Watchman (Boston Scientific, Marlborough, MA, USA), are discussed. Recently introduced devices, such as the LAmbre (Lifetech Scientific Co, Ltd, Shenzhen, China) or the Ultraseal (Cardia, Eagan, MN), are also reviewed, and finally, the new prototypes in preclinical or in the initial clinical stage are summarized[1,2] (Table 1).

ENDOCARDIAL APPROACH

Amplatzer Cardiac Plug and Amplatzer Amulet

The Amplatzer devices (Amulet and Amplatzer Cardiac Plug) are self-expanding devices with a distal lobe and a proximal disc connected by an articulated waist. The devices are made of a nitinol mesh with 2 polyester patches sewn onto the 2 components. The devices are retrievable and repositionable, and they are implanted from the femoral vein using a transeptal approach.

The Amulet device is an evolution of the Amplatzer Cardiac Plug, and it was introduced in 2012 and obtained the CE mark in January 2013. Despite the similarity in design compared with the Amplatzer Cardiac Plug,[3–6] the Amulet had several novelties, including

---

Disclosure Statement: Dr I. Cruz-Gonzalez is proctor and consultant for Abbott Vascular and Boston Scientific. Dr Y. Y. Lam is proctor for LAmbre Left Atrial Appendage Occluder.

[a] Cardiology Department, University Hospital of Salamanca, Biomedical Research Institute of Salamanca (IBSAL), CIBER-CV, Paseo San Vicente, Salamanca 37007, Spain; [b] Cardiology Department, Centre Medical, 62 Mody road, East Tsim Sha Tsui, Hong Kong, China

* Corresponding author. Cardiology Department, University Hospital of Salamanca, Paseo San Vicente 58-182, Salamanca 37007, Spain.

E-mail address: i.cruz@usal.es

Intervent Cardiol Clin 7 (2018) 253–265
https://doi.org/10.1016/j.iccl.2017.12.011

Table 1
Descriptive summary of the main devices of closure of left appendage

	Amplatzer Amulet	Watchman	LAmbre	Ultraseal	Coherex WaveCrest	Lariat
Design	Distal lobe and proximal disc	Parachute-shaped device	Umbrella and a cover connected with a short central waist	Proximal disc and a distal lobe	Umbrella shape and distal anchoring	Percutaneous epicardial LAA ligation guided by an endocardial magnet tipped wire placed in the LAA
Sizes lobe	8 sizes (16, 18, 20, 22, 25, 28, 31, and 34 mm)	5 sizes (21, 24, 27, 30, and 33 mm)	11 sizes (16, 18, 20, 22, 24, 26, 28, 30, 32, 34, and 36 mm)	9 sizes (16, 18, 20, 22, 24, 26, 28, 30, and 32 mm)	3 sizes (22, 27, and 32 mm)	Maximum target size: W 40 × H 20 × L 70 (Lariat+: W 45)
Sheaths	12–14F	14F	8–10F	10–12F	12F	12F Lariat suture delivery device
Device selection	3–6 mm longer than LAA neck diameter	10%–20% longer than LAA neck diameter	3–8 mm longer than the measured LAA orifice	Bulb diameter at least 25% to 33% greater than the largest diameter of the landing zone	The smaller device size is chosen so that the longest measured diameter does not exceed the nominal device size and the average of the longest and shortest diameters is at least 3 mm below the nominal device size	Not applicable

(Courtesy of Amulet image courtesy of Abbott Vascular, IL; Watchman image courtesy of Boston Scientific, Burlington, MA; LAmbre image courtesy Lifetech Scientific Co, Ltd, Shenzhen, China; Ultraseal image courtesy of Cardia, Eagan, MN; Coherex WaveCrest System image courtesy of Coherex Medical, Biosense Webster, Johnson & Johnson, Salt Lake City, UT; LARIAT device image courtesy of SentreHEART, Redwood City, CA; with permission.)

the following: (1) device preloaded system, (2) increased number of stabilizing wires (6–10 pairs), (3) inverted attaching end-screw on the disc, (4) larger available sizes (31 mm and 34 mm), (5) longer lobe length (7.5–10 mm), (6) longer connecting waist (5.5–8 mm), and (7) the proximal disc diameter, which is 6 or 7 mm larger than that of the lobe (compared with 4 or 6 mm with Amplatzer Cardiac Plug) depending on the size of the device (Fig. 1).

Amulet devices are usually implanted using the double curved TorqVue 45° x 45° sheath. Twelve-French sheaths are used for devices with sizes 16, 18, 20, 22, and 25 mm. Fourteen-French sheaths are selected for devices with sizes 28, 31, and 34 mm. Amulet sizing is based on the maximum left atrial appendage (LAA) landing zone (between 10 and 12 mm from the ostium), and this should be ≥11 mm and less than 31 mm.

Device deployment technique and signs of stability have been previously described[7,8] (Fig. 2).

Initially, most of the data for the Amplatzer Cardiac Plug device was derived from small registries maintained at centers outside the United States. However, a pooled analysis of 1047 procedures performed in 22 centers outside the United States[9] was published in 2016. The complication rate was 4.97%. Death, stroke, transient ischemic attack, cardiac tamponade, major bleeding, and device embolization were 0.76%, 0.86%, 0.38%, 1.24%, 1.24%, and 0.77%, respectively.

The results of the global, prospective Amplatzer Amulet observational study have been recently published.[10] This registry documents real-world periprocedural, transesophageal echocardiogram (TEE), and clinical outcomes using the Amplatzer Amulet device (n = 1088 patients). Successful device implantation was achieved in 99.0% of patients. During the procedure and index hospitalization, major adverse events occurred in 3.2% of patients, and TEE follow-up after the procedure showed adequate (<3-mm jet) occlusion of the appendage in 98.2% of patients.

The Amplatzer Amulet LAA Occluder trial (Amulet IDE) started enrolling patients in August 2016, randomizing patients in a 1:1 fashion to either the Amulet device or the Watchman device. The purpose is that the Amule device will be evaluated for safety and efficacy by demonstrating its performance is noninferior to Watchman in patients with nonvalvular atrial fibrillation in order to obtain US Food and Drug Administration (FDA) approval. The primary safety endpoint is a composite of procedure-related complications or all-cause death or major bleeding through 12 months, and the primary efficacy endpoint is a composite of ischemic stroke or systemic embolism through 18 months.

From the authors' experience, the Amulet device is versatile and a complete device that can fit in almost any LAA anatomy. It can cover from ≥11 mm to less than 31 mm (landing zone), and only 10- to 12-mm minimum depth is needed to deploy the device. It can be especially useful in chicken-wing anatomies and in the presence of thrombus.[8,11]

Watchman Left Atrial Appendage Device

The current Watchman LAA Closure Technology consists of a parachute-shaped device with a

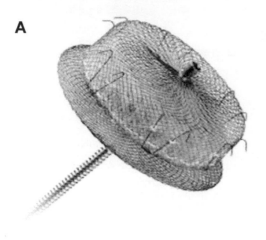
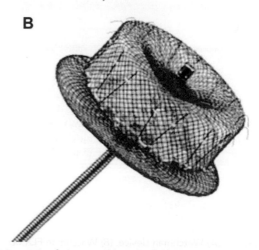

Fig. 1. (A) Amplatzer Cardiac Plug. (B) Amplatzer Amulet. (*Courtesy of* Abbott, Abbott Park, IL; with permission.)

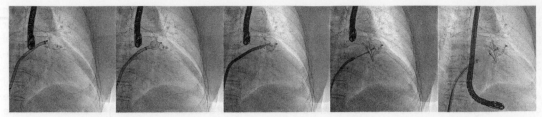

Fig. 2. Amulet device (Abbott Vascular) deployment (see text for a detailed explanation). (*Courtesy of* Abbott, Abbott Park, IL; with permission.)

self-expanding nitinol frame structure with a permeable polyester membrane (polyethylene terephthalate [PET]) over the left atrial surface. There are 10 active fixation anchors at the nitinol frame perimeter, designed to engage LAA tissue for device stability (Fig. 3A).

The device is available in 5 sizes (21, 24, 27, 30, and 33 mm) and is delivered through dedicated 14F sheaths with 12F inner diameter and 75-cm working length. Watchman sizing is based on the maximum LAA ostium diameter, which should be 17 to 31 mm to accommodate available devices. Oversizing is recommended by 9% to 25% based on the widest measurement (Fig. 4).

The Watchman FLX was the newest generation of Watchman device[12,13] introduced on November 2015 in Europe. The Watchman FLX device was similarly a self-expanding nitinol frame structure with fixation anchors and a PET fabric cover. It had several new features compared with the previous generation: (1) it was available in 5 sizes (20, 24, 27, 31, and 35 mm) for ostia measuring from 15 mm to 32 mm in width, (2) it had a reduced device length, (3) the proximal face was flat, (4) the nitinol 18-strut frame (compared with the 10-strut frame in the previous version) provided 80% more contact points at the LAA ostium, (5) atraumatic closed distal end had a fluoroscopic marker, (6) 12 "J"-shaped fixation anchors in 2 rows created a proximal and distal line to aid in device stabilization, (7) a greater range of compression was allowed, ranging from 10% to 27% (Fig. 3B).

However, at the end of March 2016, Boston Scientific decided to withdraw Watchman FLX devices because of a higher-than-anticipated device embolization rate.

From the authors' personal experience (not reported), the Watchman FLX was a very interesting device with a few new features that made its manipulation, deployment, and release easier than the old versions of Watchman. The high rate of embolization could be a combination of deployment technique and technical aspects of the device itself (distribution and angulation of anchors, range of compression permitted, and so on). A new version of the FLX is expected for 2018.

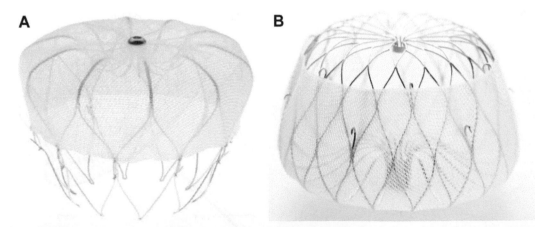

Fig. 3. (*A*) Watchman device. (*B*) Watchman FLX occluder. (Image provided *courtesy of* Boston Scientific. ©2018 Boston Scientific Corporation or its affiliates. All rights reserved.)

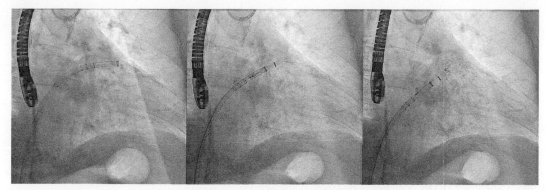

Fig. 4. Watchman device (Boston Scientific) implantation (see text for a detailed explanation). (Image provided *courtesy of* Boston Scientific. ©2018 Boston Scientific Corporation or its affiliates. All rights reserved.)

The Watchman device has been extensively studied, including the randomized, prospective, and multicenter PROTECT-AF (WATCHMAN Left Atrial Appendage System for Embolic Protection in Patients With Atrial Fibrillation) trial,[14–16] the PREVAIL (Prospective Randomized Evaluation of the WATCHMAN LAA Closure Device in Patients With Atrial Fibrillation vs Long-Term Warfarin Therapy),[17] and the recently published Registry on Watchman Outcomes in Real-Life Utilization (EWOLUTION).[18–20]

LAmbre

The LAmbre device (Lifetech Scientific Co, Ltd, Shenzhen, China) has recently obtained the CE mark on 15 June 2016. It is a nitinol-based, self-expanding device comprising a hook-embedded umbrella and a cover connected with a short central waist (Fig. 5). The waist acts as an articulating, compliant connection between the cover and the umbrella, allowing the cover to self-orient to the cardiac wall. The cover is 4 to 6 mm larger in diameter than the umbrella; however, there are devices available with a cover 12 to 14 mm larger than the umbrella (these devices could be useful for small LAA with wide orifices or for LAA with multiple shallow lobes). The proximal cover is filled with sewn-in PET. The distal umbrella comprises 8 claws with individual stabilizing hooks attaching. The umbrella was specially engineered to allow for complete collapse and repositioning. An additional PET membrane was introduced to the umbrella in the newer version of the implant to ensure LAA sealing (Fig. 6). Several sizes of the implants (16–36 mm) have been developed to accommodate the variation of LAA anatomy, and they are delivered by sheaths that ranged from 8 to 10 French in size.

The size of the implant should be 4 to 8 mm larger than the measured LAA orifice. The delivery sheath containing the implant is placed on the proximal part of the LAA. The umbrella is partially deployed by slowly pushing the device out from the delivery sheath. The whole system is then gently pushed forward to the desired landing zone to allow better flowering of the umbrella and grasping of LAA walls by the retention hooks. The sheath is then withdrawn to expose the disc, allowing it to expand in the left atrium and covering the LAA ostium by gently pushing the delivery cable forward.

Gentle tug test by applying tension to the delivery cable is performed to ensure device stability. The implant can be intentionally recaptured, completely retrieved, and redeployed. The first evidence of its efficacy and safety has been already published.[21–23] Larger trials are currently underway (eg, Study of Safety and Efficacy of a Left Atrial Appendage

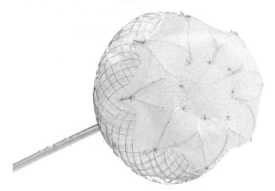

Fig. 5. LAmbre device (Lifetech Scientific Co, Ltd) consisting of a fabric-enriched cover and an umbrella connected by a short central waist. (*Courtesy of* Lifetech Scientific Co, Ltd, Shenzhen, China; with permission.)

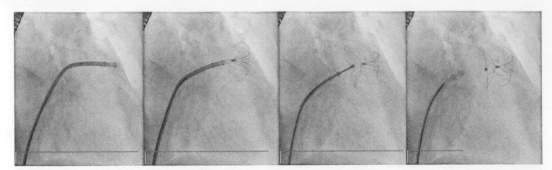

Fig. 6. LAmbre device (Lifetech Scientific Co, Ltd) implantation (see text for a detailed explanation). (*Courtesy of* Lifetech Scientific Co, Ltd, Shenzhen, China; with permission.)

Occluder; NCT02937025), and the launch of a 3-year global postmarket surveillance study has been recently announced. This registry plans to enroll more than 500 patients from about 30 clinical centers in Europe, Asia, and South America.

From the authors' limited personal experience,[22,23] this device is highly adaptable to different LAA morphologies, and it can be very useful in difficult anatomies. The combination of distal hooks and the U-shaped ends and the central waist design may help to achieve complete sealing and to prevent embolization in complex cases. Furthermore, the distal aspect of umbrella is covered by PET membrane, and this characteristic could make this device suitable for LAA occlusion with thrombus (the covered umbrella could potentially prevent thrombus migration).[24]

Ultraseal

The Ultraseal LAA closure device (Cardia, Eagan, MN, USA) obtained the CE mark in 2016; it is a self-expandable device composed of 3 parts (Fig. 7): (1) a distal bulb that anchors the device into the LAA, (2) a proximal sail that occludes the LAA, and (3) an articulating center post that connects those sections at the central portion of the device frame. The struts, which provide the structure of the device, are made of stranded nitinol. The distal bulb has 12 hooks that prevent dislodgment of the device from the appendage. The hooks are held by a radiopaque collar.

The device is available in 9 different bulb sizes ranging from 16 mm to 32 mm. The seal diameter is 6 mm larger than the distal bulb, and delivery sheath sizes range from 10F to 12F.

The landing zone for the anchoring hooks of the device should be measured at a depth of 10 to 12 mm from the intended seal location. The selected device should have a bulb diameter at least 25% to 33% greater than the largest diameter of the landing zone.

The steps for implanting the device are as follows: (1) the distal end of the sheath should be positioned in the LAA at the intended landing zone, (2) holding the sheath in place, the forceps are advanced until the entire bulb section of the device is deployed, (3) the sheath is retracted until the entire seal section of the device is deployed (Fig. 8).

Regueiro and colleagues[25] and Sabiniewicz and colleagues[26] published their experience in 2016 with the Ultraseal device in 12 patients and 6 patients, respectively. The device was successfully implanted in most patients without any major periprocedural complication.

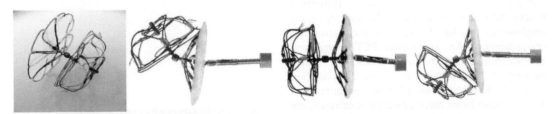

Fig. 7. Ultraseal LAA device (Cardia) consists of proximal disc and a distal lobe connected by a double articulating center for optimal positioning and repositioning within the appendage. (*Courtesy of* Cardia, Eagan, MN; with permission.)

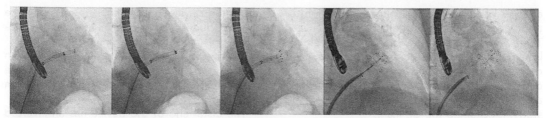

Fig. 8. Ultraseal (Cardia) implantation (see text for a detailed explanation). (*Courtesy of* Cardia, Eagan, MN; with permission.)

From the authors' limited personal experience, the articulating joint of this device allows a significant amount of movement in multiple directions in order to conform to the variations of LAA anatomy. It can be especially useful in LAA with a tight angle at the level of the landing zone or for chicken-wing anatomies.

The Coherex WaveCrest System

The Coherex WaveCrest (Coherex Medical, Biosense Webster, Johnson & Johnson, Salt Lake City, UT, USA) is a device with an umbrella shape. The device is anchored with 20 microtines distributed circumferentially at the distal device margin. The occluder material is expanded polytetrafluoroethylene (ePTFE). It is available in 3 sizes (22 mm, 27 mm, 32 mm). It is deployed similarly to other endovascular devices and has been tested in animals and humans with satisfactory and promising results. The delivery sheath is inserted just distal to the landing zone and rotated in alignment with the neck. Deployment is a 2-step procedure: unsheathing the foamed leading edge cover and then rolling out the distal anchors. At the end of each step, position and orientation of the device are confirmed on contrast angiography and TEE images.

The device was first implanted in June 2012. In 2015, the design was refined as follows (generation 1.3 device): (1) additional and optimized anchors were added, (2) increased ePTFE coverage, (3) redesigned threads and ergonomics improve closure and ease of use (Fig. 9).

The Coherex WAVECREST I Left Atrial Appendage Occlusion Study (NCT02239887) conducted in Europe, Australia, and New Zealand enrolled 73 patients with the current-generation device, and it was completed in 2015. Forty-five-day data showed primary

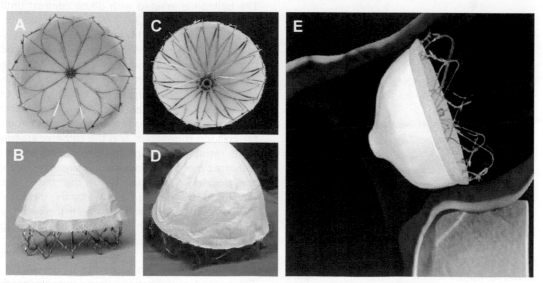

Fig. 9. The Coherex WaveCrest System. (*A*, *B*) First version device. (*C*, *D*) New design (2015 year) with additional anchors and more ePTFE covage. (*E*) Device deployment: sheath is placed in the LAA ostium and retracted to deploy the occluder. Anchors are then advanced to fix the occluder. (*Courtesy of* Coherex Medical, Salt Lake City, UT; with permission.)

efficacy of 92% and 97% with an intention-to-treat and as-treated protocol, respectively. There were no procedural strokes, device embolization, or device-associated thrombus, and only 2.7% had major adverse events (2 pericardial effusions requiring percutaneous drainage and 1 major bleeding event). As a result of this study, it obtained the CE mark.

Recently, the recruitment phase of the WAVECREST PMCF Study (NCT03204695) has started. It is a prospective, nonrandomized, multicenter study to confirm safety and performance of the Coherex WaveCrest in the current medical practice setting. The primary outcome measures are the incidence of all-cause deaths and device- and/or procedure-related events (45 days) and the secondary outcome measures: rate of successful device release within LAA, technical success at implant, and procedural.

OTHER ENDOCARDIAL DEVICES

There are more devices in development with limited clinical experience so far.

The LAA Occluder Occlutech (Occlutech International, Helsingborg, Sweden) consists of a self-expanding, flexible nitinol mesh. It has a tapered cylindrical shape that adapts to the shape of the LAA (Fig. 10). The proximal part has a larger diameter to seal the orifice. The loops at the distal rim aid in keeping the

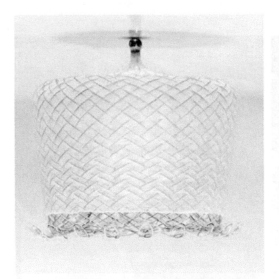

Fig. 10. Occlutech LAA (Occlutech International) occlusion device is a flexible nitinol-based, self-expanding device consisting of an outer surface covered with a nonwoven, biostable poly(carbonate) urethane layer. (*Courtesy of* Occlutech International, Helsingborg, Sweden; with permission.)

implanted device in position. The outer surface of the occluder is covered with a nonwoven, biostable poly(carbonate) urethane layer.

The size of the LAA closure device was chosen according to the LAA landing zone with a device size (diameter of distal part) about 3 to 5 mm oversized.

The distal end of the device has an inverted floor to reduce elongation during deployment and enhance anchoring stability.[27]

Occlutech won CE mark approval in the European Union for its LAA occluder device in June 2016. However, during both the LAA trial and commercial use, 4 dislocations were reported, so that the company has suspended for the moment shipping and selling of the occluder.

The Sideris Patch or The Transcatheter Patch (Custom Medical Devices, Athens, Greece) is a frameless, balloon-deliverable device used for the occlusion of heart defects. This device is bioabsorbable and can be adjusted for the shape and size of the LAA. The patches are tailored from polyurethane foam. The supporting balloon is made from latex and is inflated to diameters of 15 to 25 mm by diluted contrast. A 2-mm nylon loop is sutured at the bottom of the patch, to which a double nylon thread is connected for retrieval purposes. It is attached by a 2-stage polyethylene glycol surgical adhesive that is applied to the distal half of the device. Activation of the adhesive is achieved by direct injection of alkaline solution.

The device complex is advanced through the long sheath over the guidewire into the LAA. The balloon is inflated with dilute contrast until it stretches the LAA (3–10 mL of injectable volume corresponds to 14- to 25-mm patch diameter). Subsequently, alkaline solution is injected through the central lumen of the catheter. The balloon/patch position is confirmed by fluoroscopy and TEE. The supportive balloon catheter is removed 45 minutes after surgical adhesive activation according to the following procedure: the balloon is deflated, and the catheter assembly is retracted through the introducing sheath with the tip of the sheath held against the patch; the position and stability of the patch are confirmed by pulling lightly on the retrieval thread under echocardiography. If the result is satisfactory, the patch is released by removing the double nylon thread.

This device was studied in 20 patients showing successful placement in 17 cases.[28] There was 1 complication related to the procedure; namely, thrombus was released from the long sheath in the left atrium upon withdrawal and required treatment to be dissolved. No recurrent strokes were reported. The Transcatheter Patch has CE mark approval for the use of occlusion of heart defects in general.

An improved version of the Sideris Patch is the Prolipsis device, tested in 10 patients with good acute outcomes (full occlusion, no embolization, no pericardial effusion, no thrombosis) and long-term follow-up (full occlusions, no new strokes or stroke-related deaths).

The LeFort device (Shape Memory Alloy Co, Shangai, China) is a new-design dedicated LAA device, consisting of a self-expanding nitinol frame covered with permeable PET membrane and 10 active fixation anchors. LeFort LAA occlusion plug was designed as an umbrella-shaped device with a size of 21 mm to 33 mm consisting of nickel titanium alloy metal stent outside and the flow-barrier inside. The metal stent was covered by a polyester synthetic fiber membrane on the upper part and a protruding barbule on the lower part.[29]

SeaLA LAA Occluder (Hangzhou Nuomao Medtech Co, Zhejiang, China) is a new occluder device designed as an umbrella shaped device. It consists of one seal disc and one anchor disc and a flexible connection between them. It has a nitinol braiding mesh for the whole device that helps to adapt different LAA anatomic structures. The seal disc consists of one plate and one waist, and 3 PET membranes are sutured inside. There are 9 hooks around the outer surface of the anchor disc. The device is delivered through an 8F to 10F sheath. Preclinical studies have revealed the SeaLA LAA Occluders' safety and feasibility in canines. The China FDA and CE Clinical Studying will be used to further evaluate its safety and feasibility.

Numerous next-generation LAA closure technologies are in various stages of development and clinical testing as is PFM device (PFM Medical, Köln, Germany).

EPICARDIAL APPROACH

Epicardial approaches offer advantages of avoiding the need for transeptal puncture, risk of acute procedure-related thromboembolism, and device embolism.[30]

Sierra Ligation System or AEGIS system (Aegis Medical, Vancouver, British Columbia, Canada) permits LAA closure via epicardial approach and has 3 major components: a deflectable sheath, a deflectable grabber, and the hollow suture stiffened with a preloaded 0.25-mm wire (Fig. 11). This device introduces an appendage grabber, via percutaneous subxiphoid pericardial access, with embedded electrodes within the jaws permitting electrical navigation onto the appendage via bipolar electrograms that identify the electrical activity of the tissue captured by the jaws. A hollow suture preloaded with a support wire to permit remote suture loop manipulation and fluoroscopic visualization is advanced to the appendage base and looped around the appendage. The loop can be variably sized to accommodate multiple LAA lobes and shapes. Following loop closure, the wire is removed leaving only suture behind, which is remotely locked with a clip to maintain closure.[31] A small series has demonstrated feasibility in humans.[32]

Recently, Aegis Medical Innovations Inc has received Investigational Testing Authorization approval from Health Canada to initiate a clinical trial called LASSO-AF in Canada for this device.

The AtriClip LAA Occlusion System (AtriCure, Mason, OH, USA) is a clip made of 2 parallel rigid titanium tubes with elastic nitinol springs covered with a knit-braided polyester sheath (Fig. 12) and is placed epicardially at the base of the appendage. For human use, the clip is available in 4 sizes (35 mm, 40 mm, 45 mm, and 50 mm). When closed, the clip applies uniform pressure over the length of the 2 parallel branches to ensure occlusion of the LAA.

There are several published series of its use in humans,[33,34] the largest included 71 patients undergoing open cardiac surgery at 7 US centers. The left atrial appendage in 1 patient was too small and did not meet eligibility criteria; the remaining 70 patients had successful placement of the device. Intraprocedural successful left atrial appendage exclusion was confirmed in 67 of 70 patients (95.7%). Although significant adverse events occurred in 34 of 70 patients (48.6%), there were no adverse events related to the device and no perioperative mortality. At 3-month follow-up, 1 patient died and 65 of 70 patients (92.9%) were available for assessment. Of the patients who underwent imaging, 60 of 61 patients (98.4%) had successful LAA exclusion by computed tomography angiography or TEE imaging.[35] The Atriclip is the only FDA-approved surgical device for LAAO.

HYBRID APPROACH

The LARIAT system (SentreHEART, Redwood City, CA, USA) uses percutaneous epicardial LAA ligation guided by an endocardial magnet-

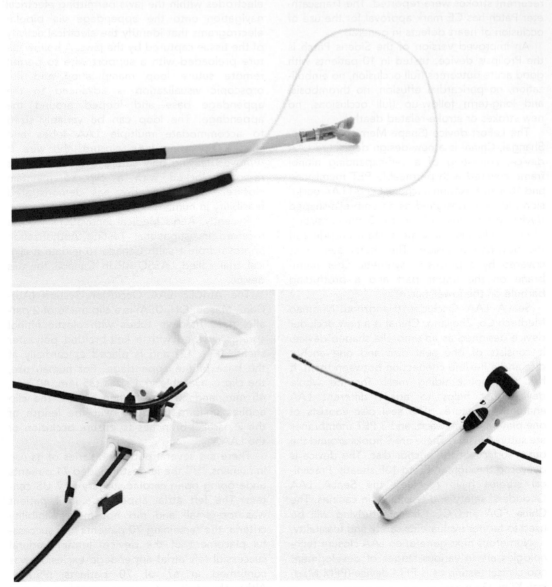

Fig. 11. Sierra ligation system. (*Courtesy of* Aegis Medical, Vancouver, British Columbia, Canada; with permission.)

tipped wire placed in the LAA via the transseptal approach, with a second magnet-tipped wire placed epicardially in union to form a rail over which an epicardial suture loop is advanced and then closed. An endocardial balloon at the LAA ostium defines where the epicardial suture needs to be placed (Fig. 13).

After initial human reports,[36] the experience in a series of 89 patients has been reported with successful closure in 85 patients (96%). A subsequent report of 27 patients with AF and high stroke risk unable to take anticoagulants, acute success was seen in 25 patients with TEE-confirmed persistent closure at 4 months

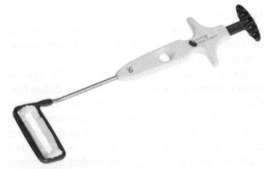

Fig. 12. The AtriClip device. (*Courtesy of* AtriCure, Mason, OH; with permission.).

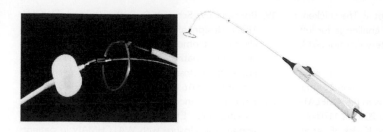

Fig. 13. LARIAT device. (*Courtesy of* SentreHEART, Redwood City, CA; with permission.)

in 22 patients.[37] Complications included LAA perforation (n = 1), pericarditis (n = 3), transseptal sheath thrombus causing stroke (n = 1), and late cerebrovascular accident (n = 1). The LARIAT has CE mark approval for commercial use. The LARIAT system device is approved by the FDA for soft tissue closure (approximation) only, but not specifically for prevention of thromboembolism with LAA occlusion. In July 2015, the FDA issued a safety communication stating that cases of death and complications such as perforation of the heart or complete LAA detachment from the heart associated with the use of LARIAT had been reported. These real-world data raised concerns about the procedural safety of this device.

The next-generation Lariat for LAA ligation (The LARIAT+) has already implanted in 58 patients and published the experience recently, with acceptably low periprocedural adverse events.[38] The new design has improved features consisting of the following: (1) expansion of the snare from 40 mm to 45 mm, (2) addition of a platinum-iridium "L" Marker that allows one for easier identification of the correct orientation of the LARIAT + snare loop under fluoroscopy, (3) a stainless steel wire braid on catheter shaft that provides improved "torque-ability" of the catheter with 1:1 torque control for ease of positioning during LAA capture.

FUTURE PERSPECTIVE

Percutaneous LAA occlusion devices represent a safe and effective therapeutic option to reduce the stroke burden in patients with nonvalvular AF.

The current results of LAAO show a high success rate with a low rate of complications. The newer generations of the most used devices and the new devices currently under development seek to be able to adapt to any type of atrial left appendage morphology (eg, small appendages, tight angle at the level of the landing zone, or complex morphologic variants), with high success rates of implantation and a decrease in the rate of major complications during the

procedure and in the long-term follow-up, as well as offer a complete coverage of the LAA that translates into a low clinical event. The new materials used for the sealing should allow a rapid endothelialization of the device that translates into a low thrombogenesis on its surface. Clinical studies are needed not only to compare their efficacy against the new oral anticoagulants but also to compare the superiority of one over the other and not to attribute a class effect of closure superiority (percutaneous, surgical, or hybrid) on anticoagulant treatment in the prevention of ischemic stroke.

REFERENCES

1. Betts TR, Leo M, Panikker S, et al. Percutaneous left atrial appendage occlusion using different technologies in the United Kingdom: a multicenter registry. Catheter Cardiovasc Interv 2017;89(3): 484–92.
2. Saw J, Lempereur M. Percutaneous left atrial appendage closure: procedural techniques and outcomes. JACC Cardiovasc Interv 2014;7(11): 1205–20.
3. Lam SC, Bertog S, Gafoor S, et al. Left atrial appendage closure using the Amulet device: an initial experience with the second generation Amplatzer Cardiac Plug. Catheter Cardiovasc Interv 2015;85(2):297–303.
4. Gloekler S, Shakir S, Doblies J, et al. Early results of first versus second generation Amplatzer occluders for left atrial appendage closure in patients with atrial fibrillation. Clin Res Cardiol 2015;104(8): 656–65.
5. Abualsaud A, Freixa X, Tzikas A, et al. Side-by-side comparison of LAA occlusion performance with the Amplatzer Cardiac Plug and Amplatzer Amulet. J Invasive Cardiol 2016;28(1):34–8.
6. Freixa X, Abualsaud A, Chan J, et al. Left atrial appendage occlusion: initial experience with the Amplatzer™ Amulet™. Int J Cardiol 2014;174(3): 492–6.
7. Tzikas A, Gafoor S, Meerkin D, et al. Left atrial appendage occlusion with the AMPLATZER Amulet device: an expert consensus step-by-step approach. EuroIntervention 2016;11(13):1512–21.

8. Freixa X, Tzikas A, Basmadjian A, et al. The chicken-wing morphology: an anatomical challenge for left atrial appendage occlusion. J Interv Cardiol 2013; 26(5):509–14.

9. Tzikas A, Shakir S, Gafoor S, et al. Left atrial appendage occlusion for stroke prevention in atrial fibrillation: multicentre experience with the AMPLAT-ZER cardiac plug. EuroIntervention 2016;11:1170–9.

10. Landmesser U, Schmidt B, Nielsen-Kudsk JE, et al. Left atrial appendage occlusion with the AMPLAT-ZER Amulet device: periprocedural and early clinical/echocardiographic data from a global prospective observational study. EuroIntervention 2017;13(7):867–76.

11. Tarantini G, D'Amico G, Latib A, et al. Percuta-neous left atrial appendage occlusion in patients with atrial fibrillation and left appendage thrombus: feasibility, safety and clinical efficacy. EuroIntervention 2017. [Epub ahead of print].

12. Grygier M, Olasińska-Wiśniewska A, Araszkiewicz A, et al. The Watchman FLX – a new device for left atrial appendage occlusion – design, potential benefits and first clinical experience. Postepy Kardiol Inter-wencyjnej 2017;13(1):62–6.

13. Seeger J, Birkemeyer R, Rottbauer W, et al. First experience with the Watchman FLX occluder for percutaneous left atrial appendage closure. Cardi-ovasc Revasc Med 2017;18(7):512–6.

14. Holmes DR, Reddy VY, Turi ZG, et al, PROTECT AF Investigators. Percutaneous closure of the left atrial appendage versus warfarin therapy for prevention of stroke in patients with atrial fibrillation: a rando-mised non-inferiority trial. Lancet 2009;374(9689): 534–42.

15. Reddy VY, Holmes D, Doshi SK, et al. Safety of percutaneous left atrial appendage closure: results from the watchman left atrial appendage system for embolic protection in patients with AF (PROTECT AF) clinical trial and continued access registry. Circulation 2011;123:417–24.

16. Reddy VY, Doshi SK, Sievert H, et al, PROTECT AF Investigators. Percutaneous left atrial appendage closure for stroke prophylaxis in patients with atrial fibrillation: 2.3-year follow-up of the PROTECT AF (Watchman Left Atrial Appendage System for Embolic Protection in Patients with Atrial Fibrilla-tion) trial. Circulation 2013;127:720–9.

17. Holmes DR Jr, Kar S, Price MJ, et al. Prospective randomized evaluation of the Watchman left atrial appendage closure device in patients with atrial fibrillation versus long-term warfarin therapy: the PREVAIL trial. J Am Coll Cardiol 2014;64:1–12.

18. Boersma LV, Schmidt B, Betts TR, et al, EWOLU-TION Investigators. Implant success and safety of left atrial appendage closure with the WATCHMAN device: periprocedural outcomes from the EWO-LUTION registry. Eur Heart J 2016;37(31):2465–74.

19. Boersma LV, Schmidt B, Betts TR, et al. EWOLU-TION: design of a registry to evaluate real-world clinical outcomes in patients with AF and high stroke risk-treated with the WATCHMAN left atrial appendage closure technology. Catheter Cardio-vasc Interv 2016;88(3):460–5.

20. Boersma LV, Ince H, Kische S, et al, EWOLUTION Investigators. Efficacy and safety of left atrial appendage closure with WATCHMAN in patients with or without contraindication to oral anticoagu-lation: 1-year follow-up outcome data of the EWO-LUTION trial. Heart Rhythm 2017;14(9):1302–8.

21. Lam YY. A new left atrial appendage occluder (Lifetech LAmbre Device) for stroke prevention in atrial fibrillation. Cardiovasc Revasc Med 2013;14:134–6.

22. Cruz-Gonzalez I, Moreno-Samos JC, Rodriguez-Collado J, et al. Percutaneous closure of left atrial appendage with complex anatomy using a Lam-bre device. JACC Cardiovasc Interv 2017;10(4): e37–9.

23. Cruz-González I, Freixa X, Fernández-Díaz JA, et al. Left atrial appendage occlusion with the Lambre device: initial experience. Rev Esp Cardiol (Engl Ed) 2017 [pii:S1885-5857(17)30219-0].

24. Cruz-Gonzalez I, Fuertes Barahona M, Moreno-Samos JC, et al. Left atrial appendage occlusion in the presence of thrombus with a Lambre device. JACC Cardiovasc Interv 2017;10(21):2224–6.

25. Regueiro A, Bernier M, O'Hara G, et al. Left atrial appendage closure: initial experience with the Ultraseal device. Catheter Cardiovasc Interv 2017; 90(5):817–23.

26. Sabiniewicz R, Hiczkiewicz J, Wańczura P, et al. First-in-human experience with the Cardia Ultraseal left atrial appendage closure device: the feasibility study. Cardiol J 2016;23(6):652–4.

27. Kim JS, Lee SG, Bong SK, et al. Preclinical assess-ment of a modified Occlutech left atrial appendage closure device in a canine model. Int J Cardiol 2016;221:413–8.

28. Toumanides S, Sideris EB, Agricola T, et al. Trans-catheter patch occlusion of the left atrial appendage using surgical adhesives in high-risk patients with atrial fibrillation. J Am Coll Cardiol 2011;58:2236–40.

29. Li S, Zhu M, Lu Y, et al. Overlay technique for trans-catheter left atrial appendage closure. Heart Lung Circ 2015;24(8):e133–5.

30. Blackshear JL, Johnson WD, Odell JA, et al. Thoracoscopic extracardiac obliteration of the left atrial appendage for stroke risk reduction in atrial fibrillation. J Am Coll Cardiol 2003;42(7): 1249–52.

31. Friedman PA, Asirvatham SJ, Dalegrave C, et al. Percutaneous epicardial left atrial appendage closure: preliminary results of an electrogram

guided approach. J Cardiovasc Electrophysiol 2009;20(8):908–15.

32. Bruce CJ, Asirvatham SJ, McCaw T, et al. Novel percutaneous left atrial appendage closure. Cardiovasc Revasc Med 2013;14(3):164–7.

33. Salzberg SP, Plass A, Emmert MY, et al. Left atrial appendage clip occlusion: early clinical results. J Thorac Cardiovasc Surg 2010;139(5):1269–74.

34. Starck CT, Steffel J, Emmert MY, et al. Epicardial left atrial appendage clip occlusion also provides the electrical isolation of the left atrial appendage. Interact Cardiovasc Thorac Surg 2012;15(3):416–8.

35. Ailawadi G, Gerdisch MW, Harvey RL, et al. Exclusion of the left atrial appendage with a novel device: early results of a multicenter trial. J Thorac Cardiovasc Surg 2011;142(5):1002–9, 1009.e1.

36. Bartus K, Bednarek J, Myc J, et al. Feasibility of closed-chest ligation of the left atrial appendage in humans. Heart Rhythm 2011;8(2):188–93.

37. Stone D, Byrne T, Pershad A. Early results with the LARIAT device for left atrial appendage exclusion in patients with atrial fibrillation at high risk for stroke and anticoagulation. Catheter Cardiovasc Interv 2015;86(1):121–7.

38. Bartus K, Gafoor S, Tschopp D, et al. Left atrial appendage ligation with the next generation LARIAT(+) suture delivery device: early clinical experience. Int J Cardiol 2016;215:244–7.

Left Atrial Appendage Occlusion, Shared Decision-Making, and Comprehensive Atrial Fibrillation Management

Michael H. Hoskins, MD[a], Anshul M. Patel, MD, FHRS[b],
David B. DeLurgio, MD, FHRS[b],*

KEYWORDS

• Left atrial appendage occlusion • Shared decision-making • Atrial fibrillation

KEY POINTS

• The epidemic of atrial fibrillation (AF) requires a comprehensive management strategy that uses the full force of available data and technology, including anticoagulation, ablative therapy, and left atrial appendage occlusion.
• Patient-centered care with an emphasis on shared decision-making is particularly relevant to the authors' understanding of the complexity of AF and has helped them tailor therapy in this ever-growing patient population.

INTRODUCTION

Case Example

A 70-year-old woman with hypertension and diabetes fell while walking her dog 6 months ago and suffered a moderate traumatic subdural hematoma. Surgical evacuation was successful, and the patient has since returned to normal activity. Two months ago she developed intermittent palpitations, and an event recorder detected paroxysms of atrial fibrillation (AF). She was treated with beta blockade and a class Ic agent. She is now referred to discuss stroke risk-reduction options.

AF has become a worldwide epidemic.[1] The complexities of AF management have grown with the prevalence of the condition, driven by growing understanding of AF pathophysiology and morbidity and improved treatment options, including new oral anticoagulants, catheter ablation, and left atrial appendage occlusion (LAAO). In this article, the authors discuss the roles of anticoagulation and LAAO in comprehensive AF management in the context of patient-centered care and shared decision-making (SDM).

THE BALANCE BETWEEN STROKE AND BLEEDING RISK IN ATRIAL FIBRILLATION

The risk of stroke and systemic embolism is increased in AF by approximately 5-fold.[1,2] Based on population studies and stroke registries, AF is implicated in up to 33% of cases.[3,4] Cardio-embolism from the left atrial appendage (LAA) is the likely source, and these events tend to be more disabling because of the potential for a large clot burden.[5] Anticoagulation by vitamin K antagonism reduces the risk of stroke.

Potential Conflicts of Interest: Abbott Medical: minor; speaking fees, research support (M.H. Hoskins). Abbott Medical: minor; speaking fees, research support (A.M. Patel). Abbot Medical, Boston Scientific: minor; speaking fees, research support, consultant (D.B. DeLurgio).

[a] Emory University School of Medicine, Emory University Hospital, 1364 Clifton Road Northeast, Suite F424, Atlanta, GA 30322, USA; [b] Emory University School of Medicine, Emory St. Joseph's Hospital, 5671 Peachtree Dunwoody Road, Suite 300, Atlanta, GA 30342, USA
* Corresponding author.
E-mail address: ddelurg@emory.edu

2211-7458/18/© 2017 Elsevier Inc. All rights reserved.

More recently, direct oral anticoagulants (DOACs), including a direct thrombin inhibitor and 3 factor Xa inhibitors, have also been approved in patients with nonvalvular AF.[6–9]

Stroke Risk in Atrial Fibrillation

Treatment with a vitamin K antagonists (VKAs) or DOACs in AF is based on the estimated stroke risk. Risk stratification schemes help guide a decision to anticoagulate. The most widely used are the $CHADS_2$ (congestive heart failure, hypertension, age, diabetes, stroke or transient ischemic attack) and, more recently, CHA_2DS_2-VASc scores. In the $CHADS_2$ score, congestive heart failure (1 point), hypertension (1 point), age greater than 75 years (1 point), diabetes (1 point), and stroke or transient ischemic attack (TIA) (2 points) are taken

into account. A score of 2 or greater is an indication for anticoagulation with warfarin. The CHA_2DS_2-VASc score adds moderate risk factors like age greater than 65 years (1 point), female sex (1 point), and vascular disease or previous myocardial infarction (MI) (1 point) and gives an additional point for age greater than 75 years (2 points). Similarly, a score of 2 or greater is an indication for anticoagulation (Fig. 1).

The risk of stroke using these scores has been validated and generally increases with the accumulation of risk factors.[10,11] For example, a $CHADS_2$ score of 1 gives an annual stroke risk of 3.4%, whereas a score of 4 gives about an 8.9% annual stroke risk. The initial validation cohort for the $CHADS_2$ score showed a high correlation with stroke risk.[10] However, its

Risk Factors	SCORE
Congestive heart failure	1
Hypertension	1
Age 75 or greater	2
Age 65–74	1
Diabetes Mellitus	1
Stroke/TIA/systemic embolism	2
Vascular disease	1
Sex (female)	1
Your score	

CHA_2DS_2-VASc Score	ADJUSTED STROKE RATE (% per year)
0	0% or very low
1	1.3%
2	2.2%
3	3.2%
4	4.0 %
5	6.7%
6	9.8%
7	9.6%
8	6.7%
9	15.2%

Fig. 1. CHA_2DS_2-VASc and HAS-BLED stroke and bleeding risk scores and associated annual risk of stroke or bleeding events. CHA_2DS_2-VASc stroke risk score. (*Adapted from* Pisters R, Lane DA, Nieuwlaat R, et al. A novel user-friendly score [HAS-BLED] to assess 1-year risk of major bleeding in patients with atrial fibrillation: the Euro Heart Survey. Chest 2010;138:1096; with permission.)

performance in later cohorts with lower-risk patients, such as the Anticoagulation and Risk Factors in Atrial Fibrillation (ATRIA) and Euro Heart Survey, showed a much less reliable correlation.[12]

CHA_2DS_2-VASc was developed to overcome the shortcomings of the $CHADS_2$ score.[11] The stroke risk based on CHA_2DS_2-VASc is outlined in Fig. 1. A particular strength of the CHA_2DS_2-VASc score lies in its ability to identify those patients in a low-risk category (score = 0) who should not be treated with anticoagulation. It is also better at risk stratifying patients who would have had a $CHADS_2$ score of 0 but still carry a risk of stroke that can be up to 3.8% per year.[13] It is now the guideline standard for determining the stroke risk and need for anticoagulation.[14,15]

A common misconception is that paroxysmal AF carries a lower stroke risk than persistent or permanent AF. However, epidemiologic data suggest the stroke risk is similar.[16] Patients with atrial flutter should also be considered for stroke prophylaxis. The most recent European and American guidelines recommend all patients with AF and atrial flutter be considered for anticoagulation if their stroke risk score is elevated.

Anticoagulation and Atrial Fibrillation

The efficacy of anticoagulation for stroke prophylaxis in AF is undisputed. Warfarin was the established therapy for more than 30 years. Meta-analyses of the original trials comparing warfarin with placebo showed a 39% to 64% reduction in stroke and systemic embolism.[17] Even more recent data show that anticoagulation can reduce the risk of stroke from approximately 4% to 1%, which is similar to matched controls without AF.[18] In a recent meta-analysis, warfarin reduced the stroke risk to 1.66%, with a mean time in the therapeutic range of 62.6%.[19] However, real world treatment with VKAs is challenged by issues with dosing, drug interactions, international normalized ratio (INR) monitoring, and compliance.

DOACs are increasingly prescribed, particularly in anticoagulation-naïve patients. They have more predictable dosing and fewer drug interactions. A meta-analysis of all 4 DOAC trials versus warfarin confirmed an approximately 19% stroke risk reduction with similar rates of bleeding (except gastrointestinal [GI]) and dramatic reductions in intracranial hemorrhage (ICH) versus warfarin.[20] There was also a 10% all-cause mortality reduction

(Table 1). Warfarin is still the drug of choice for patients with mechanical heart valves, rheumatic valve disease, and in those with chronic kidney disease. In addition, aspirin should not be offered as stroke prophylaxis in AF.[21] In the AVERROES study, apixaban had similar rates of major bleeding and ICH to aspirin but with significantly better stroke reduction.[22]

Bleeding Risk on Anticoagulation

Lifelong anticoagulation increases bleeding risk, and this remains the leading therapeutic obstacle. Assessing bleeding risk is an important component of AF management. There is a variety of scores that have been published, including the HAS-BLED, $HEMORR_2HAGES$, and ATRIA bleeding risk scores.[23–25] The easiest to use and best validated is the HAS-BLED score. It uses clinical predictors, including uncontrolled hypertension, renal disease, liver disease, previous stroke, labile INRs, previous bleeding event, use of nonsteroidal antiinflammatory drugs or antiplatelet agents, age greater than 65 years, and alcohol use. Each risk factor carries equal weighting (1 point). A score of 3 or higher is considered high risk (Fig. 2). Even though bleeding is a consideration, it is generally recommended to not withhold anticoagulation even in those with high HAS-BLED scores, as they are often the ones who benefit the most. For one large cohort of 13,559 patients, the benefit of anticoagulation when the bleeding risk was taken into consideration was still 0.68% and even higher (~2.0%) in patients with a previous history of stroke or the elderly.[26]

The most dreaded complication of anticoagulation is ICH, which includes intraparenchymal bleeds, subdural hematomas, and subarachnoid hemorrhage. The annual rate of ICH on warfarin in one large pooled analysis was 0.61%.[16] It seems that anticoagulation-associated ICH is more morbid. Interestingly, DOACs reduce the risk of ICH versus warfarin with an estimated risk reduction of 0.44.[17] Generally, rapid reversal of anticoagulation for ICH is recommended. For VKAs, this usually includes administering fresh frozen plasma, vitamin K, and even activated factor VIIa. Reversibility of anticoagulation has been perceived as an advantage of warfarin over the DOACs. However, there is now a Food and Drug Administration (FDA)–approved reversal agent for dabigatran called idaracuzimab.[27] There are also published data on a reversal agent for factor Xa inhibitors called adexenet alpha.[28]

Table 1
Comparison of warfarin and direct oral anticoagulants in major clinical trials

	Dabigatran (RE-LY)	Rivaroxaban (ROCKET-AF)	Apixaban (ARISTOTLE)	Edoxaban (Engage AF-TIMI 48)
Mechanism	Oral direct thrombin inhibitor	Oral direct factor Xa inhibitor	Oral direct factor Xa inhibitor	Oral direct factor Xa inhibitor
Bioavailability (%)	6	66 fasting 80–100 with food	50	62
Time to peak levels (h)	3	2–4	3	1–2
Half-life (h)	12–17	5–13	9–14	10–14
Excretion	80% renal	66% liver, 33% renal	27% renal	50% renal
Dosage	150 mg twice daily or 110 mg twice daily	20 mg once daily	5 mg twice daily	60 mg once daily or 30 mg once daily
Dosage reduction in selected patients	—	Rivaroxaban 15 mg once daily if creatine clearance 30–49 mL/min	Apixaban 2.5 mg twice daily if at least 2 y ≥80 y, body weight ≤60 kg, or serum creatinine level ≥1.5 mg/dL (133 μmo/L)	Edoxaban 60 mg reduced to 30 mg once daily, and edoxaban 30 mg reduced to 15 mg once daily, if any of the following: creatinine clearance of 30–50 mL/min, body weight ≤60 kg, concomitant use of verapamil or quinidine or dronedarone
Study design	Randomized, open label	Randomized, double blind	Randomized, double blind	Randomized, double blind
Number of patients	18,113	14,264	18,201	21,105
Follow-up period (y)	2.0	1.9	1.8	2.8
Randomized groups	Dose-adjusted warfarin vs blinded doses of dabigatran (150 mg twice daily, 110 mg twice daily)	Dose-adjusted warfarin vs rivaroxaban 20 mg once daily	Dose-adjusted warfarin vs apixaban 5 mg twice daily	Dose-adjusted warfarin vs edoxaban (60 mg once daily, 30 mg once daily)
Age (y)	71.5 ± 8.7 (mean ± SD)	73 (65–78) (median [interquartile range])	70 (63–76) (median [interquartile range])	72 (64–78) (median [interquartile range])
Male sex (%)	63.6	60.3	64.5	61.9
CHADS$_1$ score (mean)	2.1	3.5	2.1	2.8

	Warfarin n = 6022 Event Rate (%)/y	Dabigatran 150 n = 6076 Event Rate (%)/y (RR vs Warfarin)	Dabigatran 110 n = 6015 Event Rate (%)/y (RR vs Warfarin)	Warfarin n = 7133 Event Rate (%)/y	Rivaroxaban n = 7131 Event Rate (%)/y (HR vs Warfarin)	Warfarin n = 9081 Event Rate (%)/y	Apixaban n = 9120 Event Rate (%)/y (HR vs Warfarin)	Warfarin n = 7036 Event Rate (%)/y	Edoxaban 60 n = 7035 Event Rate (%)/y (HR vs Warfarin)	Edoxaban 30 n = 7034 Event Rate (%)/y (HR vs Warfarin)
Stroke/systemic embolism	1.72	1.12 (0.65, 0.52–0.81; P for non inferiority and superiority <.001)	1.54 (0.89, 0.73–1.09; P for non inferiority <.001)	2.4	2.1 (0.88, 0.75–1.03; P for non inferiority <.001, P for superiority = .12)	1.60	1.27 (0.79, 0.66–0.95; P<.001 for non inferiority, P = .01 for superiority)	1.80	1.57 (0.87, 0.73–1.04; P<.001 for non inferiority, P = .08 for superiority)	2.04 (1.13, 0.96–1.34; P = .05 for non inferiority, P = .10 for superiority)
Ischemic stroke	1.22	0.93 (0.76, 0.59–0.97; P = .03)	1.34 (1.10, 0.88–1.37; P = .42)	1.42	1.34 (0.94; 0.75–1.17; P = .581)	1.05	0.97 (0.92, 0.74–1.13; P = .42)	1.25	1.25 (1.00, 0.83–1.19; P = .97)	1.77 (1.41, 1.19–1.67; P<.001)
Hemorrhagic stroke	0.38	0.10 (0.26, 0.14–0.49; P<.001)	0.12 (0.31, 0.17–0.56; P<.001)	0.44	0.26 (0.59; 0.37–0.93; P = .024)	0.47	0.24 (0.51, 0.35–0.75; P<.001)	0.47	0.26 (0.54, 0.38–0.77; P<.001)	0.16 (0.33, 0.22–0.50; P<.001)
Major bleeding	3.61	3.40 (0.94, 0.82–1.08; P = .41)	2.92 (0.80, 0.70–0.93; P = .003)	3.45	3.60 (1.04; 0.90–2.30; P = .58)	3.09	2.13 (0.69, 0.60–0.80; P<.001)	3.43	2.75 (0.80, 0.71–0.91; P<.001)	1.61 (0.47, 0.41–0.55; P<.001)
Intracranial bleeding	0.77	0.32 (0.42, 0.29–0.61; P<.001)	0.23 (0.29, 0.19–0.45; P<.001)	0.74	0.49 (0.67; 0.47–0.93; P = .002)	0.80	0.33 (0.42, 0.30–0.58; P<.001)	0.85	0.39 (0.47, 0.34–0.63; P<.001)	0.26 (0.30, 0.21–0.43; P<.001)
GI major bleeding	1.09	1.60 (1.48, 1.19–1.86; P<.001)	1.13 (1.04, 0.82–1.33; P = .74)	1.24	2.00 (1.61; 1.30–1.99; P<.001)	0.86	0.76 (0.89, 0.70–1.15; P = .37)	1.23	1.51 (1.23, 1.02–1.50; P = .03)	0.82 (0.67, 0.53–0.83; P<.001)
MI	0.64	0.81 (1.27, 0.94–1.71; P = .12)	0.82 (1.29, 0.96–1.75; P = .09)	1.12	0.91 (0.81; 0.63–1.06; P = .12)	0.61	0.53 (0.88, 0.66–1.17; P = .37)	0.75	0.70 (0.94, 0.74–1.19; P = .60)	0.89 (1.19, 0.95–1.49; P = .13)
Death from any cause	4.13	3.64 (0.88, 0.77–1.00; P = .051)	3.75 (0.91, 0.80–1.03; P = .13)	2.21	1.87 (0.85, 0.70–1.02; P = .07)	3.94	3.52 (0.89, 0.80–0.99; P = .047)	4.35	3.99 (0.92, 0.83–1.01; P = .08)	3.80 (0.87, 0.79–0.96; P = .006)

Abbreviations: HR, hazard ratio; RR, relative risk.

Clinical Characteristic	SCORE
Hypertension	1
Abnormal liver function	1
Abnormal renal function	1
Stroke	1
Bleeding	1
Labile INRs	1
Elderly (Age greater than 65)	1
Drugs	1
Alcohol	1
Your score	

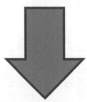

HAS-BLED Score	BLEEDING RISK (% per year)
0	0.9
1	3.4
2	4.1
3	5.8
4	8.9
5	9.1

Fig. 2. HAS-BLED score.

The decision to resume anticoagulation after ICH is individualized based on the relative risk of rebleeding and stroke and is best done in consultation with neurology and/or neurosurgery. There are little data to guide safety. If resumed, a DOAC may be preferred given their more favorable risk profile.

GI bleeding is very common on warfarin.[29–31] In general, randomized controlled trials and meta-analyses have suggested that the GI bleeding risk for the DOACs may be slightly higher than warfarin; but there are differences between the agents. For example, in the RE-LY trial, dabigatran 110 mg had similar GI bleeding to warfarin, whereas dabigatran 150 mg had a higher rate. In ARISTOTLE, GI bleeding between warfarin and apixaban were similar. In the trial for edoxaban, the low dose (30 mg) had similar bleeding risks to warfarin and the higher dose (60 mg) had more GI bleeding. In ROCKET-AF, which was a higher-risk population, there were 8 more bleeding events per 1000 patients annually versus warfarin[6–8,30,32] (see Table 1). Reversal of anticoagulation in GI bleeding may be less urgent than in ICH, particularly if patients are hemodynamically stable and can be transfused appropriately. In general, the anticoagulation should be withheld acutely. Resuming it again depends on the severity of the bleed and how definitive treatment was of the source of bleeding.[33] Unfortunately, bleeding remains an issue with all anticoagulant agents.

LAAO devices (eg, Watchman, Boston Scientific Corporation, St Paul, MN, Amulet, Abbott Medical, St Paul, MN) have been developed as an alternative to anticoagulation for stroke prophylaxis in AF. In the PROTECT-AF trial, long-term follow-up at a mean of 3.8 years showed that the Watchman device was superior to warfarin for the primary outcome of stroke, systemic embolism, and cardiovascular death. It also met superiority criteria for cardiovascular and all-cause mortality.[34] Placing these devices avoids the need for long-term anticoagulation and, thus, reduces the risk of bleeding. It also does not rely on patient compliance, which is another major factor in determining the effectiveness of treatment.

THE INTERSECTION OF LEFT ATRIAL APPENDAGE OCCLUSION AND ATRIAL FIBRILLATION ABLATION

Utilization of ablation therapy for the treatment of symptomatic AF has increased dramatically, and emerging clinical data are beginning to establish the safety and efficacy of combining LAAO and catheter ablation for AF. However, the concept of using these two strategies in tandem is not novel. In fact, the Cox-maze series of ablation techniques involves ligation of the LAA in part as an attempt to reduce the risk of future stroke.[35] The contemporary revisiting of this model using a catheter-based approach represents a reconvergence of 2 techniques, which had previously been on separate paths of development. The ability to perform 2 technically separate, if not pathophysiology distinct, procedures highlights the importance of approaching AF comprehensively. With this combined strategy, there is potential to reduce both symptoms of arrhythmia and stroke risk with a single nonsurgical procedure.

Several issues arise when considering patients who potentially need catheter ablation and LAAO for AF. These issues include the anatomic proximity of the LAA to the pulmonary veins, the effect of ablation on or near an LAAO device, the role of the LAA in arrhythmogenesis, and the need for oral anticoagulation (OAC) after ablation in patients who may be poor candidates for these medications. In addition, whether to perform these procedures simultaneously or sequentially is an important consideration.

COMBINED ABLATION/LEFT ATRIAL APPENDAGE OCCLUSION: REVIEW OF THE DATA

In 2012, Swaans and colleagues[36] described the feasibility of a combined procedure. This study included 30 patients with a mean $CHADS_2$ score of 2.5. Patients underwent radiofrequency catheter ablation followed immediately by LAAO with the Watchman device. All patients had successful LAAO device implantation. Follow-up Transesophageal echocardiography (TEE) data showed no peri-device leaks, and no thromboembolic events occurred at 1 year.

Other groups have subsequently evaluated the safety and efficacy of concomitant radiofrequency ablation/LAAO procedures.[37–39] These cohorts have been relatively small (35–98 patients), and most of the patients received Watchman devices (185 Watchman, 10 Amplatzer, Abbott, St Paul, Minnesota). Acute LAAO success was excellent (97%–100%). The arrhythmia recurrence rate during follow-up (mean of 38 months) ranged from 22% to 42%, which is comparable with the accepted stand-alone ablation procedure data. Major complications, bleeding, pericardial effusions, stroke, and death, were infrequent. Follow up TEE data identified satisfactory LAAO in 95-100% of patients (including peri-device leaks < 5 mm).

Heeger and colleagues[40] evaluated the effect of radiofrequency catheter ablation of left atrial arrhythmias in 8 patients who had previously undergone LAA closure (7 Watchman, 1 Amplatzer). These patients all underwent pulmonary vein isolation, with some patients also receiving linear ablation or ablation of complex fractionated atrial electrograms. The patients had a mean $CHADS_2$-$VASC_2$ score of 3.6 ± 0.7 and had ablation performed a mean of 201 (range 41–746) days after LAAO. No acute interaction with the LAAO device and the ablation catheter was seen, and no thrombus was seen on TEE 1 day after ablation. One patient developed a thrombus on the Watchman device on follow-up TEE performed 112 days after ablation, despite being actively treated with dabigatran. This thrombus persisted for 616 days after treatment with various novel anticoagulants. The authors, therefore, recommend careful follow-up assessment with TEE after this approach.

Turagam and colleagues[41] performed a larger retrospective analysis of 60 patients undergoing catheter ablation after previously having LAAO with the Watchman device. Twenty-eight percent of patients in the cohort had LAA triggers. This study showed that, although radiofrequency ablation was safe and feasible in these patients, isolation of the LAA with a Watchman device present was challenging, with only a modest success rate (62%). Importantly, 10% of patients developed new significant leaks (>5 mm) and subsequently required extension of the period during which they were treated with anticoagulation.

Fassini and colleagues[42] evaluated the simultaneous use of catheter ablation with cryoablation and LAAO. This study included 35 patients with AF (80% paroxysmal) undergoing pulmonary vein isolation with cryo-balloon ablation. All patients underwent LAAO following ablation. Twenty-five patients underwent Watchman implantation, and 10 patients underwent Amplatzer Cardiac Plug implantation. In all patients, LAAO was successful, with 5 patients demonstrating an acute peri-device leak (<5 mm) at implant. The addition of LAAO to cryo-balloon ablation added 9 ± 3 minutes of fluoroscopy and 44 ± 12 minutes of procedural time. No acute or subacute thrombus formation was detected on TEE, and no clinical thromboembolic events were seen at the 1-year follow-up.

ROLE OF LEFT ATRIAL APPENDAGE IN ARRHYTHMOGENESIS: CONSIDERATIONS FOR LEFT ATRIAL APPENDAGE OCCLUSION

The LAA is increasingly recognized as a potential trigger for atrial arrhythmias.[43,44] In one series of patients with AF, the LAA was found to be the trigger in 27% of patients. Electrical isolation of the LAA has been described using both radiofrequency[45] and cryo-ablation[46] techniques. Although isolation of the LAA has been shown to increase the effectiveness of catheter ablation for AF, there is evidence this may increase the stroke risk by promoting thrombus formation within a mechanically inactive appendage.[47] Furthermore, endovascular closure of the LAA (ie, with Watchman or Amplatzer devices) may subsequently inhibit the ability to adequately record LAA signals or effectively achieve electrical isolation. Thus, the concept of combining electrical and mechanical isolation of the LAA is appealing as a means to reduce the risk of stroke while eliminating a potential trigger for arrhythmia.

Epicardial ligation of the LAA with the Lariat device (SentreHEart, Palo Alto, CA) has been shown to decrease LAA electrical activity[48] and reduce AF burden in patients with long-term monitoring devices.[49] This effect may be more prominent in patients with persistent AF and in those with known LAA triggers. The addition of LAAO with the Lariat device plus catheter ablation has been shown in an observational study to decrease the recurrence of AF and need for repeat procedures in patients with persistent AF.[50] An ongoing clinical trial is evaluating the effectiveness of LAA ligation

with the Lariat device as an adjunct to catheter ablation as a means to reduce arrhythmia recurrence (clinicaltrials.com NCT02513797). The increasing understanding of the role of the LAA in arrhythmogenesis in addition to stroke underscores the importance of careful selection and timing of LAAO for an individual patient.

TECHNICAL CONSIDERATIONS FOR PATIENTS UNDERGOING BOTH CATHETER ABLATION AND LEFT ATRIAL APPENDAGE OCCLUSION

The technical considerations when performing catheter ablation and LAAO depend in part on whether the procedures are performed simultaneously or sequentially. When performed simultaneously, the LAAO portion of the procedure has typically been performed after ablation. This practice adds procedural and fluoroscopy time as well as the use of contrast. In addition, although some centers use conscious sedation for catheter ablation, LAAO procedures typically require the use of general anesthesia and continuous TEE guidance. Finally, although standard anticoagulation regimens after LAAO include only 6 weeks of OAC (or perhaps none at all), current expert consensus[51] recommends at least 2 months of OAC after catheter ablation.

Although catheter ablation for AF is widely used in most electrophysiology laboratories, the insertion of LAAO devices (in the United States) requires several additional mandates. These mandates include the need for a shared decision discussion and minimum CHADS$_2$-VASc$_2$ scores and may limit the ability to perform simultaneous procedures in some patients.

When catheter ablation is performed after prior LAAO, several additional considerations arise. The proximity of the LAAO device to the pulmonary veins may prove technically challenging when ablating along the ridge between the LAA and the left pulmonary veins. This challenge may be more of an issue with the Amplatzer device, which has a disk that extends along a portion of the limbus. In addition, the biophysical interaction between these devices and radiofrequency or cryoablation energy is not well described. There is at least one report of thrombus forming on the surface of an LAAO after ablation was performed.[40] The rate of ablation-related device leaks may be unacceptably high as well.[41,42] Finally, the role of the LAA as a trigger or substrate for AF may not be evident at the time of LAAO, and the presence of an occluder device may inhibit the ability to adequately ablate this area at a later date. The complex role of the LAA and surrounding anatomy in the genesis of AF lends support to the concept of a comprehensive approach. Accordingly, the authors' recommendation is that electrophysiologists be involved in the decision tree for the management of these patients.

MANAGEMENT OF ANTICOAGULATION AFTER LEFT ATRIAL APPENDAGE OCCLUSION

Oral Anticoagulation After Watchman

Management of OAC after LAAO may differ depending on which product is used. Adjustment of medications after the Watchman procedure has been outlined in the PROTECT-AF and PREVAIL trials.[52,53] Patients are typically prescribed aspirin 81 mg daily as well as warfarin (goal INR 2–3) for 45 days after the implant. If the follow-up TEE shows adequate seal and no device-associated thrombus, warfarin is discontinued and patients start aspirin (81–325 mg daily) and clopidogrel (75 mg daily) for the remainder of the 6 months. At 6 months after the implant, patients transition to indefinite aspirin. If the 45-day postimplant TEE shows thrombus and/or leak greater than 5 mm, repeat TEE is recommended at 6 months after the implant. Patients should continue OAC during this time or until the leak or thrombus resolves.

In the ASAP trial,[54] patients who were deemed unable to tolerate short-term OAC were prescribed only antiplatelet therapy after the Watchman implant. This therapy consisted of clopidogrel 75 mg for 6 months after the implant as well as aspirin indefinitely. The observed ischemic stroke rate in this trial was 1.7% per year, which compared favorably with historical controls based on the risk of enrolled patients. A randomized controlled trial comparing aspirin and clopidogrel use versus Watchman with aspirin/clopidogrel combination therapy is currently enrolling for patients unable to tolerate short-term OAC (clinicaltrials.gov NCT02928497).

A recently published registry evaluated 1025 patients who were prospectively evaluated after the Watchman procedure.[55] In this real-world experience, anticoagulation regimens included VKAs (16%), novel OACs (NOACs) (11%), dual antiplatelet therapy (60%), single antiplatelet therapy (7%), or no therapy (6%). No difference in stroke was seen between these groups.

Oral Anticoagulation After Amplatzer/Amulet

The Amplatzer Cardiac Plug (ACP) and Amulet devices are based on a structural extrapolation of the Amplatzer family of atrial septal closure devices. Therefore, they have a precedent for being used without the use of OAC. Berti and colleagues[56] evaluated 110 patients who were unable to tolerate short-term OAC and who underwent implantation of either the first- (ACP) or second-generation (Amulet) Amplatzer Cardiac Plug with antiplatelet therapy. This study showed an annual stroke rate of 2.2% per year in a patient population with a mean $CHADS_2\text{-}VASc_2$ score of 4.3. The currently enrolling Amulet trial allows investigators to use either dual antiplatelet therapy for 6 months followed by aspirin therapy indefinitely or a regimen similar to that used for the Watchman device (clinicaltrials.gov NCT02879448).

Oral Anticoagulation After Lariat

Limited comparative data exist for the use of OAC or antiplatelet therapy alone for the Lariat device. The lack of any endovascular structure requiring endothelialization offers the theoretic advantage of not requiring OAC.[57] A minimum of antiplatelet therapy is typically used with the Lariat device, but further data are required for understanding the need for anticoagulation with this technology.

Novel Anticoagulants After Left Atrial Appendage Occlusion

The use of NOACs after LAAO is an appealing strategy for several reasons, including ease of use, rapid time to therapeutic activity, and the relatively short period of time that patients are expected to remain on OAC after LAAO. Enomoto and colleagues[58] retrospectively evaluated 214 patients treated with NOACs after LAAO and compared them with a control cohort receiving warfarin. Ninety-two percent of these patients were on either rivaroxaban or apixaban, and most (82%) continued NOAC therapy uninterrupted through the LAAO procedure. The rate of peri-procedure bleeding complications was the same in both groups (1.9%), and one patient in each group experienced either a stoke or TIA. In addition, the rate of device-associated thrombus was low in each group (0.9% for NOAC, 0.5% for warfarin). These data suggest that NOACs offer a safe, effective, and simple way to anticoagulate patients in the immediate postprocedure period after LAAO.

POSTPROCEDURE IMAGING

The role of imaging after LAAO is to assess device positioning and evaluate for device-associated thrombus and peri-device leaks. Considerations include timing and modality of imaging. TEE remains the mainstay for most centers, benefiting from ease of interpretation and consistency with the protocols in clinical trials. In the PROTECT-AF and PREVAIL trials, TEE was performed at 45 days, 6 months, and 12 months after the implant. Combined cohorts from PROTECT-AF and CAP demonstrated a rate of device-associated thrombus of 4.2%, and an additional evaluation of the PROTECT-AF cohort demonstrated a rate of thrombus of 5.7%.[59]

The rate of peri-device leak after the Watchman implant was found to be 32% in the PROTECT-AF cohort[60] and 25% in another similar-sized cohort.[61] The impact of smaller leaks is debatable, and leaks as large as 5 mm in size do not seem to be associated with an increase in embolic events compared with patients without leaks. There have been no consistently identified risk factors that predict the development of leaks after the Watchman implant.

Saw and colleagues[62] performed an evaluation of follow-up TEE imaging in 605 patients who had undergone implantation with the ACP device. TEE was performed in 344 cases with a mean follow-up period of 134 days after the implant. The rate of device-associated thrombus was 3.2%, and the rate of peri-device leak was 12.5%. The presence of thrombus was treated with anticoagulation per the treating physician's opinion. None of the patients had stroke or TIA associated with thrombus. Conversely, peri-device leak was associated with stroke or TIA in 2.6% of patients.

Data regarding the presence of leaks and device-associated thrombus after the Lariat device are more limited. Pillasarti and colleagues[61] showed that the rate of peri-device leak was 2% at the time of the procedure with the Lariat device, and that increased to 25% at 45 days. There was no correlation between the presence of a leak and device-associated thrombus.

The role of computed tomography (CT) imaging after LAAO to assess for both device-associated thrombus and peri-device leak is evolving.[63,64] Berte and colleagues[63] compared TEE and CT imaging in 77 patients at 6 weeks after the implant. The rate of peri-device leak detection was comparable between the 2 imaging modalities (1.5 ± 1.9 mm vs 1.1 ± 2.1 mm, respectively). However, in 29% of patients, the degree of the peri-device leak was larger in TEE than CT; in 14% of patients, the leak was larger in CT than TEE. This discrepancy raises concern for the lack of reproducibility between the two imaging modalities, at least for relatively small leaks. One patient in this series had a device-associated thrombus noted on TEE, whereas none were reported by CT.

The authors' practice is to perform TEE at the time of LAAO and then use TEE for postprocedural imaging at 45 days and 1 year after the implant. If a device leak or thrombus is noted at 45 days, consideration for continued OAC and/or more rapid follow-up imaging is taken. This strategy has the advantage of adhering to the safety design of available clinical trials as well as offering comparative imaging during serial evaluations. CT imaging offers a noninvasive means of imaging the LAAO site, but further data are needed to confirm its utility as an appropriate stand-alone modality.

LEFT ATRIAL APPENDAGE OCCLUSION AND SHARED DECISION-MAKING

In the case example presented at the beginning of this article, it is clear that an important medical decision is in the offing. Given this patient's increased risk of thromboembolic stroke, should she begin therapy with an oral anticoagulant? Or, given her prior fall and subdural hematoma, does the risk of an anticoagulant outweigh its benefits? Is LAAO a reasonable alternative? LAAO reduces the need for long-term OAC but does require short-term anticoagulation as well as an invasive procedure. This situation lends itself well to the process of SDM, "an approach where clinicians and patients share the best available evidence when faced with the task of making decisions, and where patients are supported to consider options, to achieve informed preferences."[65] With the approval of the Watchman device for stroke risk reduction in selected patients with AF came the requirement for the inclusion of "a formal shared decision making interaction with an independent non-interventional physician using an evidence-based decision tool on oral anticoagulation in non-valvular AF prior to [LAAO]."[66] This process, an integral part of patient-centered care, is, therefore, a responsibility and mandate.

What Is Shared Decision-Making and How Do We Implement It in Left Atrial Appendage Occlusion?

The modern concept of SDM has its roots in the Presidents' Commission of 1982.[67] Although the precise definition of SDM may vary somewhat, there are 9 essential process elements described by Lin and Fagerlin[68]: (1) defining the problem, (2) presenting options, (3) discussing the risks and benefits of these options, (4) discussing patient values and preferences, (5) discussing patient ability to make decisions, (6) offering knowledge and communication, (7) checking and clarifying understanding, (8) making or deferring a decision, and (9) arranging follow-up. By carrying out this process, evidence-based medicine and communication between the health care provider and patients are effectively combined to reach a joint health care decision in full consideration of patients' specific circumstances as well as values and preferences[67].

Implementing SDM is more complex than it seems. Although the mandate for SDM exists, few physicians implement the required process elements.[69–71] Often a lack of time is cited, but a more prescient culprit is the lack of training and resources to properly conduct SDM. Despite the push for SDM using decision tools, few medical practices have access to or provide tools to conduct SDM. Tools used in SDM require scientific validation: do they achieve their goal of informing, eliciting feedback, and resulting in a shared decision? Current decision aids may include option grids,[72] figures,[73] and pictographs.[74] Web sites with decision aids for various medical conditions are available to patients and practitioners (Table 2). However, a recent systematic review found that no validated AF stroke prevention decision aids are available, and none of the published but unvalidated aids address LAAO specifically.[75–77]

What might an SDM tool for LAAO look like? In order to reach a decision between the use of an anticoagulant, a decision to forego anticoagulation, or a decision to proceed to LAAO, initially basic and then more detailed information must be presented. First, the authors find it useful to introduce the concept of thromboembolism leading to stroke in patients with AF by presenting a figure illustrating this concept (Fig. 3). The purpose of this figure and the accompanying discussion is to clearly describe the known mechanism for stroke in AF and to set the stage for the discussion of

Table 2 Internet resources for atrial fibrillation decision aids	
Organization	**Web Site**
Ottawa Hospital Research Institute	http://www.decisional aid.ohri.ca
Option grids	www.optiongrid.org
MED-DECS	http://www.med-decs.org/
Healthwise	http://www. healthwise.org
American College of Cardiology	www.acc.org/tools-and-practice-support/
National institute for Health and Care Excellence	https://ww.nice.org. uk/

the role of anticoagulation and LAAO. Next, it is important to individualize the stroke and bleeding risk to the extent possible. Because the risk of these complications varies from patient to patient, the use of the $CHADS_2$-VASc and HAS-BLED scores with the associated average annual risks is useful for patients attempting to understand their personal risk (see Figs. 1 and 2). This exchange of information is helpful in the general decision between consideration of anticoagulation versus no anticoagulation. Many patients considering LAAO have already been taking anticoagulant medication but have either experienced complications or have developed other compelling reasons to consider an alternative to long-term anticoagulant use. The authors have devised an option grid that addresses several frequently ask questions in the context of taking an anticoagulant versus proceeding to LAAO with the Watchman device (Table 3). Although this option grid has not been formally evaluated, it does help patients compare the two therapies and provide a basis for informed decision-making. Finally, the authors use a pictograph to compare 5-year outcomes with the Watchman device versus warfarin therapy (Fig. 4). This pictograph normalizes the incidence of death, hemorrhagic stroke, and ischemic stroke to a population of 1000 patients receiving either warfarin or the Watchman device. This pictograph is a useful way to present the differences in outcomes between the two options and help patients

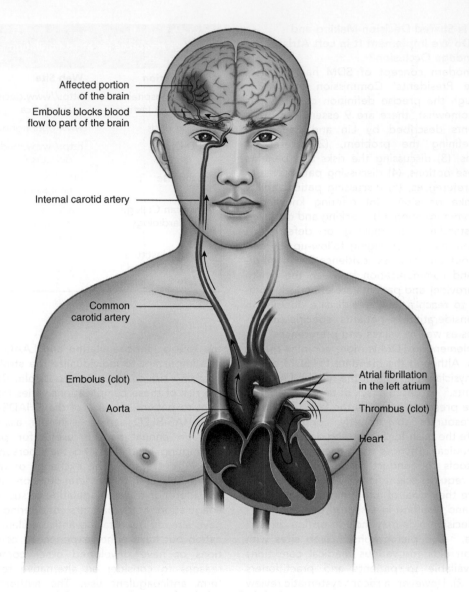

Affected portion
of the brain

Embolus blocks blood
flow to part of the brain

Internal carotid artery

Common
carotid artery

Embolus (clot)

Aorta

Atrial fibrillation
in the left atrium

Thrombus (clot)

Heart

Fig. 3. Decision aid depicting mechanism of embolic stroke linked to AF.

gauge the magnitude with regard to each outcome individually as well as combined.

The patient in the authors' clinical example has a stroke risk score of 4 and a bleeding risk score of 3. Statistically, these scores correspond to an annual stroke rate of 4% if no anticoagulant is used and an annual bleeding rate of 5.8% if warfarin is chosen. Using this information, the patient then considered LAAO with the Watchman device. Using the pictograph, she reasoned that LAAO could significantly reduce her risk of bleeding events, particularly intracranial bleeding, compared with warfarin, while still conferring the overall stroke risk reduction. She understood that an invasive procedure was involved that carried some risk; but, based on her history of requiring surgery as a result of her prior subdural hematoma, she thought this was a reasonable risk to take. She was satisfied with medical therapy for control of AF. She underwent LAAO closure with the Watchman device and discontinued warfarin 45 days later after a follow-up transesophageal echo confirmed durable LAAO.

Table 3
Option grid: warfarin/oral anticoagulation versus left atrial appendage occlusion with the Watchman device

Frequently Asked Questions	Warfarin/OAC	LAAO with Watchman Device
Is this treatment/procedure FDA approved?	Warfarin and several other newer anticoagulants are FDA approved for use in stroke risk reduction in patients with AF.	The Watchman device is FDA approved as an alternative to warfarin for stroke risk reduction.
Do I need warfarin/OAC or the Watchman Device?	The decision to use warfarin/OAC is based on individual stroke risk assessed by a stroke risk score and a discussion of risks and benefits of treatment or no treatment with a physician.	LAAO with the Watchman device may be considered as an alternative to warfarin/OAC in patients tolerant of warfarin but who have a compelling reason to consider this alternative, understanding the risks and benefits of both options.
Will treatment reduce my risk of stroke?	By thinning the blood, warfarin and the other OACs reduce the risk of clot formation within the heart that can result in a stroke. Overall, warfarin/OACs reduce the risk of stroke by 70% compared with no therapy at all. Strokes due to bleeding within the brain are more frequent and more dangerous in patients taking blood thinners.	LAAO with the Watchman device prevents the movement of clots from the heart to the brain and is as effective as warfarin in preventing this type of stroke. By reducing the need for long-term anticoagulation, the Watchman device reduces the chance of a stroke due to bleeding in the brain.
How strong is the evidence for this treatment?	The evidence for the use of warfarin/OAC is strong. The regulatory bodies state that in appropriate patients warfarin/OAC "should be considered."[15]	The evidence for LAAO closure with the Watchman device is good. The regulatory bodies state that in appropriate patients the Watchman device "may be considered."[15]
What is the risk of this treatment?	Use of warfarin/OAC is associated with an increased risk of bleeding events, both major and minor. This risk may change over time	Implantation of the Watchman device may result in surgical bleeding, either major or minor. The risk of bleeding decreases over time as blood thinning medications are eliminated.
What are reasons to consider this treatment?	Physicians may recommend warfarin/OAC in patients with AF and increased risk of stroke based on the stroke risk score. This decision involves consideration of the risks posed by the medication as well as patient preferences and values.	Physicians may recommend LAAO with the Watchman device when patients exhibit or express a compelling reason to consider an alternative to warfarin/OAC. These reasons may include bleeding events, poor toleration or compliance with warfarin/OAC, high risk of bleeding, occupational concerns, and other considerations.
What follow-up is necessary?	Patients on warfarin/OAC are seen on a regular basis to monitor response to medication. Blood work is required, more frequently for warfarin than the newer OACs.	After implantation of the Watchman device, follow-up is required at 6 wk and again at 6 mo. Long-term follow-up is not required.

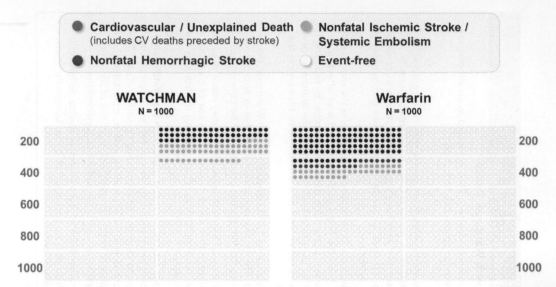

Fig. 4. Pictograph depicting outcome events for LAAO with the Watchman device versus warfarin. CV, cardiovascular.

SUMMARY

The epidemic of AF requires a comprehensive management strategy that uses the full force of available data and technology, including anticoagulation, ablative therapy, and LAAO. Patient-centered care with an emphasis on SDM is particularly relevant to the authors' understanding of the complexity of AF and has helped them tailor therapy in this ever-growing patient population.

REFERENCES

1. Kishore A, Vail A, Majid A, et al. Detection of atrial fibrillation after ischemic stroke or transient ischemic attack: a systematic review and meta-analysis. Stroke 2014;45:520–6.
2. Wolf PA, Abbott RD, Kannel WB. Atrial fibrillation as an independent risk factor for stroke: the Framingham Study. Stroke 1991;22(8):983–8.
3. Bjorck S, Palaszewski B, Friberg L, et al. Atrial fibrillation, stroke risk, and warfarin therapy revisited: a population-based study. Stroke 2013;44:3103–8.
4. Friberg L, Rosenqvist M, Lindgren A, et al. High prevalence of atrial fibrillation among patients with ischemic stroke. Stroke 2014;45:2599–605.
5. Marini C, De Santis F, Sacco S, et al. Contribution of atrial fibrillation to incidence and outcome of ischemic stroke: results from a population-based study. Stroke 2005;36(6):1115–9.
6. Connolly SJ, Ezekowitz MD, Yusuf S, et al. Dabigatran versus warfarin in patients with atrial fibrillation. N Engl J Med 2009;361(12):1139–51.
7. Patel MR, Mahaffey KW, Garg J, et al. Rivaroxaban versus warfarin in nonvalvular atrial fibrillation. N Engl J Med 2011;365(10):883–91.
8. Granger CB, Alexander JH, McMurray JJ, et al. Apixaban versus warfarin in patients with atrial fibrillation. N Engl J Med 2011;365(11):981–92.
9. Giugliano RP, Ruff CT, Braunwald E, et al. Edoxaban versus warfarin in patients with atrial fibrillation. N Engl J Med 2013;369(22):2093–104.
10. Gage BF, Waterman AD, Shannon W, et al. Validation of clinical classification schemes for predicting stroke: results from the national registry of atrial fibrillation. JAMA 2001;285:2864–70.
11. Lip GY, Nieuwlaat R, Pisters R, et al. Refining clinical risk stratification for predicting stroke and thromboembolism in atrial fibrillation using a novel risk factor-based approach: the Euro Heart Survey on Atrial Fibrillation. Chest 2010;137:263–72.
12. Keogh C, Wallace E, Dillon C, et al. Validation of the CHADS2 clinical prediction rule to predict ischaemic stroke: a systematic review and meta-analysis. Thromb Haemost 2011;106:528–38.
13. Olesen JB, Torp-Pedersen C, Hansen ML, et al. The value of the CHA2DS2-VASc score for refining stroke risk stratification in patients with atrial fibrillation with a CHADS2 score 0 – 1: a nationwide cohort study. Thromb Haemost 2012;107:1172–9.
14. Camm AJ, Lip GYH, Caterina RD, et al. 2012 focused update of the ESC guidelines for the management of atrial fibrillation. An update of the 2010 ESC guidelines for the management of atrial fibrillation. Developed with the special contribution of the European Heart Rhythm Association. Eur Heart J 2012;33:2719–47.

15. January CT, Wann LS, Alpert JS, et al. 2014 AHA/ACC/HRS guideline for the management of patients with atrial fibrillation: a report of the American College of Cardiology/American Heart Association Task Force on practice guidelines and the Heart Rhythm Society. Circulation 2014;130:e199–267.

16. Friberg L, Hammar N, Rosenqvist M. Stroke in paroxysmal atrial fibrillation: report from the Stockholm Cohort of Atrial Fibrillation. Eur Heart J 2010;31:967–75.

17. Hart RG, Pearce LA, Aguilar MI. Meta-analysis: antithrombotic therapy to prevent stroke in patients who have nonvalvular atrial fibrillation. Ann Intern Med 2007;146:857–67.

18. Freedman B, Martinez C, Katholing A, et al. Residual risk of stroke and death in anticoagulant-treated patients with atrial fibrillation. JAMA Cardiol 2016;1:366–8.

19. Agarwal S, Hachamovitch R, Menon V. Current trial-associated outcomes with warfarin in prevention of stroke in patients with nonvalvular atrial fibrillation: a meta-analysis. Arch Intern Med 2012;172:623–31.

20. Ruff CT, Giugliano RP, Braunwald E, et al. Comparison of the efficacy and safety of new oral anticoagulants with warfarin in patients with atrial fibrillation: a meta-analysis of randomised trials. Lancet 2014;383:955–62.

21. Ben Freedman S, Gersh BJ, Lip GY. Misperceptions of aspirin efficacy and safety may perpetuate anticoagulant underutilization in atrial fibrillation. Eur Heart J 2015;36:653–6.

22. Connolly SJ, Eikelboom J, Joyner C, et al. Apixaban in patients with atrial fibrillation. N Engl J Med 2011;364(9):806–17.

23. Pisters R, Lane DA, Nieuwlaat R, et al. A novel user-friendly score (HAS-BLED) to assess 1-year risk of major bleeding in patients with atrial fibrillation: the Euro Heart Survey. Chest 2010;138:1093–100.

24. Gage BF, Yan Y, Milligan PE, et al. Clinical classification schemes for predicting hemorrhage: results from the National Registry of Atrial Fibrillation (NRAF). Am Heart J 2006;151:713–9.

25. Fang MC, Go AS, Chang Y, et al. A new risk scheme to predict warfarin-associated hemorrhage: the ATRIA (Anticoagulation and Risk Factors in Atrial Fibrillation) study. J Am Coll Cardiol 2011;58:395–401.

26. Singer DE, Chang Y, Fang MC, et al. The net clinical benefit of warfarin anticoagulation in atrial fibrillation. Ann Intern Med 2009;151:297–305.

27. Pollack CV, Reilly PA, Eikelboom J, et al. Idarucizumab for dabigatran reversal. N Engl J Med 2015;373:511–20.

28. Siegal DM, Curnutte JT, Connolly SJ, et al. Andexanet alfa for the reversal of factor Xa inhibitor activity. N Engl J Med 2015;373:2413–24.

29. Lanas A, Garcia-Rodriguez LA, Polo-Tomas M, et al. Time trends and impact of upper and lower gastrointestinal bleeding and perforation in clinical practice. Am J Gastroenterol 2009;104(7):1633–41.

30. Coleman CI, Sobieraj DM, Winkler S, et al. Effect of pharmacological therapies for stroke prevention on major gastrointestinal bleeding in patients with atrial fibrillation. Int J Clin Pract 2012;66(1):53–63.

31. Holster IL, Valkhoff VE, Kuipers EJ, et al. New oral anticoagulants increase risk for gastrointestinal bleeding: a systematic review and meta-analysis. Gastroenterology 2013;145(1):105–12.e15.

32. Atrial Fibrillation Investigators. Risk factors for stroke and efficacy of antithrombotic therapy in atrial fibrillation. Analysis of pooled data from five randomized controlled trials. Arch Intern Med 1994;154:1449–57 [Erratum appears in Arch Intern Med 1994;154:2254].

33. Desai J, Granger CB, Weitz JI, et al. Novel oral anticoagulants in gastroenterology practice. Gastrointest Endosc 2013;78(2):227–39.

34. Reddy VY, Sievert H, Halperin J, et al. Percutaneous left atrial appendage closure vs warfarin for atrial fibrillation: a randomized clinical trial. JAMA 2015;313(10):1061.

35. Albage A, Sartipy U, Kenneback G, et al. Long-term risk of ischemic stroke after the Cox-maze III procedure for atrial fibrillation. Ann Thorac Surg 2017;104(2):523–9.

36. Swaans MJ, Post MC, Rensing BJ, et al. Ablation for atrial fibrillation in combination with left atrial appendage closure: first results of a feasibility study. J Am Heart Assoc 2012;1(5):1–7.

37. Alipour A, Swaans MJ, van Dijk VF, et al. Ablation for atrial fibrillation combined with left atrial appendage closure. JACC Clin Electrophysiol 2015;1(6):486–95.

38. Calvo N, Salterain N, Arguedas H, et al. Combined catheter ablation and left atrial appendage closure as a hybrid procedure for the treatment of atrial fibrillation. Europace 2015;17(10):1533–40.

39. Phillips KP, Walker DT, Humphries JA. Combined catheter ablation for atrial fibrillation and Watchman(R) left atrial appendage occlusion procedures: five-year experience. J Arrhythm 2016;32(2):119–26.

40. Heeger CH, Rillig A, Lin T, et al. Feasibility and clinical efficacy of left atrial ablation for the treatment of atrial tachyarrhythmias in patients with left atrial appendage closure devices. Heart Rhythm 2015;12(7):1524–31.

41. Turagam MK, Lavu M, Afzal MR, et al. Catheter ablation for atrial fibrillation in patients with watchman left atrial appendage occlusion device: results from a multicenter registry. J Cardiovasc Electrophysiol 2017;28(2):139–46.

42. Fassini G, Conti S, Moltrasio M, et al. Concomitant cryoballoon ablation and percutaneous closure of

left atrial appendage in patients with atrial fibrillation. Europace 2016;18(11):1705–10.

43. Di Biase L, Burkhardt JD, Mohanty P, et al. Left atrial appendage: an under-recognized trigger site of atrial fibrillation. Circulation 2010;122(2): 109–18.

44. Yamada T, McElderry HT, Allison JS, et al. Focal atrial tachycardia originating from the epicardial left atrial appendage. Heart Rhythm 2008;5(5): 766–7.

45. Di Biase L, Burkhardt JD, Mohanty P, et al. Left atrial appendage isolation in patients with long-standing persistent AF undergoing catheter ablation: BELIEF trial. J Am Coll Cardiol 2016;68(18): 1929–40.

46. Imnadze G, Kranig W, Thale J, et al. Left atrial appendage ablation using cryoballoon. Pacing Clin Electrophysiol 2017;40(11):1330.

47. Rillig A, Tilz RR, Lin T, et al. Unexpectedly high incidence of stroke and left atrial appendage thrombus formation after electrical isolation of the left atrial appendage for the treatment of atrial tachyarrhythmias. Circ Arrhythm Electrophysiol 2016;9(5):e003461.

48. Han FT, Bartus K, Lakkireddy D, et al. The effects of LAA ligation on LAA electrical activity. Heart Rhythm 2014;11(5):864–70.

49. Afzal MR, Kanmanthareddy A, Earnest M, et al. Impact of left atrial appendage exclusion using an epicardial ligation system (LARIAT) on atrial fibrillation burden in patients with cardiac implantable electronic devices. Heart Rhythm 2015;12(1):52–9.

50. Lakkireddy D, Sridhar Mahankali A, Kanmanthareddy A, et al. Left atrial appendage ligation and ablation for persistent atrial fibrillation. JACC: Clin Electrophysiol 2015;1(3):153–60.

51. Calkins H, Hindricks G, Cappato R, et al. HRS/EHRA/ECAS/APHRS/SOLAECE expert consensus statement on catheter and surgical ablation of atrial fibrillation. Heart Rhythm 2017;14(10):e275–444.

52. Holmes DR Jr, Kar S, Price MJ, et al. Prospective randomized evaluation of the Watchman left atrial appendage closure device in patients with atrial fibrillation versus long-term warfarin therapy: the PREVAIL trial. J Am Coll Cardiol 2014;64(1):1–12.

53. Reddy VY, Holmes D, Doshi SK, et al. Safety of percutaneous left atrial appendage closure: results from the Watchman Left Atrial Appendage System for Embolic Protection in Patients with AF (PROTECT AF) clinical trial and the continued access registry. Circulation 2011;123(4):417–24.

54. Reddy VY, Mobius-Winkler S, Miller MA, et al. Left atrial appendage closure with the Watchman device in patients with a contraindication for oral anticoagulation: the ASAP study (ASA Plavix feasibility study with Watchman left atrial appendage closure technology). J Am Coll Cardiol 2013;61(25):2551–6.

55. Boersma LV, Ince H, Kische S, et al. Efficacy and safety of left atrial appendage closure with WATCHMAN in patients with or without contraindication to oral anticoagulation: 1-Year follow-up outcome data of the EWOLUTION trial. Heart Rhythm 2017;14(9):1302–8.

56. Berti S, Pastormerlo LE, Rezzaghi M, et al. Left atrial appendage occlusion in high-risk patients with non-valvular atrial fibrillation. Heart 2016;102(24): 1969–73.

57. Jazayeri MA, Vuddanda V, Parikh V, et al. Percutaneous left atrial appendage closure: current state of the art. Curr Opin Cardiol 2017;32(1):27–38.

58. Enomoto Y, Gadiyaram VK, Gianni C, et al. Use of non-warfarin oral anticoagulants instead of warfarin during left atrial appendage closure with the Watchman device. Heart Rhythm 2017;14(1):19–24.

59. Main ML, Fan D, Reddy VY, et al. Assessment of device-related thrombus and associated clinical outcomes with the WATCHMAN left atrial appendage closure device for embolic protection in patients with atrial fibrillation (from the PROTECT-AF Trial). Am J Cardiol 2016;117(7): 1127–34.

60. Viles-Gonzalez JF, Kar S, Douglas P, et al. The clinical impact of incomplete left atrial appendage closure with the Watchman device in patients with atrial fibrillation: a PROTECT AF (Percutaneous Closure of the Left Atrial Appendage Versus Warfarin Therapy for Prevention of Stroke in Patients With Atrial Fibrillation) substudy. J Am Coll Cardiol 2012;59(10):923–9.

61. Pillarisetti J, Reddy YM, Gunda S, et al. Endocardial (Watchman) vs epicardial (Lariat) left atrial appendage exclusion devices: understanding the differences in the location and type of leaks and their clinical implications. Heart Rhythm 2015; 12(7):1501–7.

62. Saw J, Tzikas A, Shakir S, et al. Incidence and clinical impact of device-associated thrombus and peri-device leak following left atrial appendage closure with the Amplatzer cardiac plug. JACC Cardiovasc Interv 2017;10(4):391–9.

63. Berte B, Jost CA, Maurer D, et al. Long-term follow-up after left atrial appendage occlusion with comparison of transesophageal echocardiography versus computed tomography to guide medical therapy and data about postclosure cardioversion. J Cardiovasc Electrophysiol 2017; 28(10):1140–50.

64. Ismail TF, Panikker S, Markides V, et al. CT imaging for left atrial appendage closure: a review and pictorial essay. J Cardiovasc Comput Tomogr 2015;9(2):89–102.

65. Elwyn G, Coulter A, Laitner S, et al. Implementing shared decision making in the NHS. BMJ 2010; 341:c5146.

66. Jensen T, Chin J, Ashby L, et al. Decision memo for left atrial appendage (LAA) closure therapy (CAG-00445N). 2016. Available at: https://www.cms.gov/medicare-coverage-database/details/nca-decision-memo.aspx?NCAId=281. Accessed July 1, 2017.

67. United States. Presidents' commission for the study of ethical problems in medicine and biomedical and behavioral research. Making health care decisions: the ethical and legal implications of informed consent in the patient-practitioner relationship. U S Code Annot U S 1982;42:300v.

68. Lin G, Fagerlin A. Shared decision making: state of the science. Circ Cardiovasc Qual Outcomes 2014;7:328–34.

69. Spatz E, Spertus J. Shared decision making: a path toward improved patient-centered outcomes. Circ Cardiovasc Qual Outcomes 2012;5:e75–7.

70. Mulley A, Trimble C, Elwyn G. Stop the silent misdiagnosis: patient's preferences matter. BMJ 2012;345:e6572.

71. Elwyn G, Stiel M, Durand M, et al. The design of patient decision support interventions: addressing the theory-practice gap. J Eval Clin Pract 2011;17:565–74.

72. Elwyn G, Lloyd A, Joseph-Williams N, et al. Option grids: shared decision making made easier. Patient Educ Couns 2013;90:207–12.

73. Edwards A, Elwyn G. The potential benefits of decision aids in clinical medicine. JAMA 1999;282(8):779–80.

74. Fagerlin A, Zikmund-fisher B, Ubel P. Helping patients decide: ten steps to better risk communication. J Natl Cancer Inst 2011;103(97):1436–43.

75. O'Neill E, Grande S, Sherman A, et al. Availability of patient decision aids for stroke prevention in atrial fibrillation: a systematic review. Am Heart J 2017;191:1–11.

76. Fraenkel L, Street R, Fried T. Development of a tool to improve the quality of decision making in atrial fibrillation. BMC Med Inform Decis Mak 2011;11:59–69.

77. Eckman M, Wise R, Naylor K, et al. Developing an atrial fibrillation guideline support tool (AFGuST) for shared decision making. Curr Med Res Opin 2015;31(4):603–14.

Moving?

Make sure your subscription moves with you!

To notify us of your new address, find your **Clinics Account Number** (located on your mailing label above your name), and contact customer service at:

Email: journalscustomerservice-usa@elsevier.com

800-654-2452 (subscribers in the U.S. & Canada)
314-447-8871 (subscribers outside of the U.S. & Canada)

Fax number: 314-447-8029

Elsevier Health Sciences Division
Subscription Customer Service
3251 Riverport Lane
Maryland Heights, MO 63043

*To ensure uninterrupted delivery of your subscription, please notify us at least 4 weeks in advance of move.

ELSEVIER

Printed and bound by CPI Group (UK) Ltd, Croydon, CR0 4YY

03/10/2024

01040384-0017